Schizophrenia

YOUR QUESTIONS ANSWERED

Commissioning and Development: Fiona Conn
Project Manager: Frances Affleck
Design direction: George Ajayi

Schizophrenia

YOUR QUESTIONS ANSWERED

Trevor Turner
BA MB BS MD FRCPsych
Consultant Psychiatrist and Clinical Director, Homerton Hospital and
St Bartholomew's Hospital, London, UK

With Compliments of Eli Lilly and Company Limited

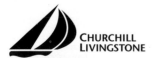

CHURCHILL
LIVINGSTONE

EDINBURGH LONDON NEW YORK OXFORD PHILADELPHIA ST LOUIS SYDNEY TORONTO 2003

CHURCHILL LIVINGSTONE
An imprint of Elsevier Science Limited

Cover image © Science Photo Library

First published 2003

ISBN 0 443 07347 3

British Library Cataloguing in Publication Data
A catalogue record for this book is available from the British Library

Library of Congress Cataloging in Publication Data
A catalog record for this book is available from the Library of Congress

Notice
Medical knowledge is constantly changing. Standard safety precautions must be followed, but as new research and clinical experience broaden our knowledge, changes in treatment and drug therapy may become necessary or appropriate. Readers are advised to check the most current product information provided by the manufacturer of each drug to be administered to verify the recommended dose, the method and duration of administration, and contraindications. It is the responsibility of the practitioner, relying on experience and knowledge of the patient, to determine dosages and the best treatment for each individual patient. Neither the Publisher nor the author assumes any liability for any injury and/or damage to persons or property arising from this publication.

 your source for books,
journals and multimedia
in the health sciences
www.elsevierhealth.com

The
publisher's
policy is to use
**paper manufactured
from sustainable forests**

Printed in China

Contents

Preface

Schizophrenia remains one of the least understood serious illnesses of today. Even though some half million patients are affected in the UK, that is to say just under 1 in 100 people, at some time in the course of their lives, it continues to be downgraded compared to cancer, heart disease, or childhood disorders. Charitable contributions to mental illness have long been niggardly compared to a range of others, reflecting the stigma attached to mental illness as a whole.

This book is designed to provide accurate information about the reality of the illness, to be clear about areas which remain uncertain, and to help GPs and families with the complex business of providing care. As with all psychiatric disorders, treatment involves a combination of pharmacological interventions, personal support with or without specialised forms of therapy, and generating a social environment that is positive and non-stigmatising. The worst consequence of modern attitudes to schizophrenia has been the notion that in some way it represents someone who is dangerous. Notions of 'Risk Management' now dominate the Government agenda, confusing Home Office and security needs with those of health and therapy. The last 30 years or more of community care have shown no evidence of any rise whatsoever in assaults or murders committed by those with psychotic illnesses, such as schizophrenia, despite the marked rise in violence committed by so-called 'normal' individuals.

The consequences of this policy approach, and the emphasis on risk, have been a creeping return to forms of asylum, patients being locked up in prisons (a rising population), high dependence hostels, forensic 'rehabilitation' units, and a range of private enterprises. Having emptied the asylums we are now fast rebuilding them, in another guise, even though most patients with schizophrenia are managed in the context of primary care.

The most important single fact about schizophrenia in the 21st century is that it is extremely treatable. We now have a range of medications, many of them only introduced in the last decade, that make it possible to remove or significantly reduce psychotic symptoms, to avoid debilitating and embarrassing side-effects, and to get people back to real social and personal lives. The main limiting factor in this is delay in initiating treatment, because of ignorance or fear of being 'labelled' as mad. Furthermore, remission is often cut short by people discontinuing medication, as often as not persuaded so to do by self-appointed gurus knowing little about the illness. Yet treatment is not just about medication nowadays. Using what is termed a 'bio-psycho-social' approach, the importance of a stable social and family environment, cognitive techniques to reduce the impact of symptoms, and the support of properly trained and organised community care terms, can all together make a real difference.

Given the prevalence of schizophrenia, on a life-time basis, the average GP will have between 10 and 20 patients on his/her books, enough to require some understanding but (obviously) not such as to require or retain specialist knowledge. This book therefore is aimed at providing succinct and therapeutically useful answers to a range of questions that may occur. The long-term nature of the illness, and its remitting/relapsing course in many individuals, can lead to a variety of types of relapse and treatment approaches. Those working regularly with schizophrenic patients also generally find them endearing, thought-provoking and strikingly honest about the psychological world in which they live.

I am indebted in producing this book to the brilliant typing and organisational skills of Jon Flint, as well as to all the colleagues, patients and families who have trusted me with their insights and support. I am also lucky to have had a most understanding associate editor, in Fiona Conn, who has nurtured this manuscript through the usual delays and complexities of NHS life.

TT

How to use this book

The *Your Questions Answered* series aims to meet the information needs of GPs and other primary care professionals who care for patients with chronic conditions. It is designed to help them work with patients and their families, providing effective, evidence-based care and management.

The books are in an accessible question and answer format, with detailed contents lists at the beginning of every chapter and a complete index to help find specific information.

ICONS
Icons are used in the book to identify particular types of information:

 highlights information important to clinical practice

 highlights side-effect information

 highlights case studies which illustrate or help to explain the answers given

PATIENT QUESTIONS
At the end of relevant chapters there are sections of frequently asked patient questions, with easy-to-understand answers aimed at the non-medical reader. These questions are also listed at the end of the book.

Historical introduction and definitions

1.1   When was schizophrenia first described?

The term 'schizophrenia' to describe a severe form of mental illness was coined by the Swiss psychiatrist Eugen Bleuler (1857–1939) and publicized in his 1911 textbook entitled *Dementia Praecox, or the group of schizophrenias.* Bleuler created the word to describe the way in which the mind seemed to be broken up in terms of its normal functioning, in that thinking, feeling and perceiving did not seem to be coherent. He also wished to get away from the negative connotations of the term 'dementia praecox' (*see Q. 1.4*), which essentially described younger people becoming thought-disordered, having delusions and hallucinations, and inevitably declining into states of self-neglect and fatuity. Schizophrenia was formulated as a means of combining the new psychoanalytic theories of Sigmund Freud (1856–1939) with the accepted descriptions of severe mental illness that were being seen in the asylums. Its definition and classification was made possible by the late-19th century diagnostic advances that enabled psychiatrists to separate out those with syphilitic brain disease, idiocy and endocrine and nutritional disorders from the mass of chronically ill, 'insane' asylum inmates. Some of the historical terms used to describe severe mental illnesses are outlined in *Figure 1.1* and Bleuler's original list of symptoms in *Table 1.1.* (*See also Ch. 3*)

1.2   What does the word 'schizophrenia' really mean?

Although the term 'schizophrenia' is constantly being misused, especially in the broadsheet press, it does *not* mean 'being in two minds', like Robert Louis Stevenson's Dr Jekyll and Mr Hyde, nor even having a split personality. The term 'schizophrenia', although derived from classical Greek ('schizo' meaning 'split' and 'phrenia' referring to 'mind' or 'mental function') was actually made up by Bleuler (*see Q. 1.1*). He considered that the 'splitting of the different psychic functions is one of [the disease's] most important characteristics'. He meant to evoke an image of the mind broken up into various parts, but influential cultural commentators (e.g. the poet and critic T.S. Eliot) took him literally, and thus was born the notion of a split mind and even two different personalities. What schizophrenia does mean is that thoughts, feelings, perceptions and beliefs do not seem to connect. It is thus a severe mental illness, with a range of characteristic symptoms, that usually comes on in a younger age group (late teens and early 20s) and tends to have a chronic or relapsing course. Furthermore, it is probably best considered as a syndrome or even a group of illnesses with different degrees of severity. The most problematic differential diagnoses

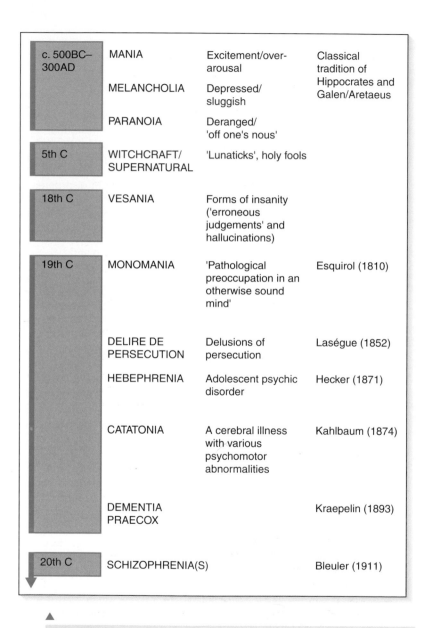

c. 500BC–300AD	MANIA	Excitement/over-arousal	Classical tradition of Hippocrates and Galen/Aretaeus
	MELANCHOLIA	Depressed/sluggish	
	PARANOIA	Deranged/'off one's nous'	
5th C	WITCHCRAFT/SUPERNATURAL	'Lunaticks', holy fools	
18th C	VESANIA	Forms of insanity ('erroneous judgements' and hallucinations)	
19th C	MONOMANIA	'Pathological preoccupation in an otherwise sound mind'	Esquirol (1810)
	DELIRE DE PERSECUTION	Delusions of persecution	Laségue (1852)
	HEBEPHRENIA	Adolescent psychic disorder	Hecker (1871)
	CATATONIA	A cerebral illness with various psychomotor abnormalities	Kahlbaum (1874)
	DEMENTIA PRAECOX		Kraepelin (1893)
20th C	SCHIZOPHRENIA(S)		Bleuler (1911)

Fig. 1.1 Historical descriptions of schizophrenia.

TABLE 1.1 Bleuler's schizophrenic symptoms 1911 (the 4 'A's)	
Primary	Ambivalence – an inability to decide or initiate things
	Autism – being self-absorbed and difficult to engage with
	Associations impaired/loosened (being unable to think coherently)
	Affect impaired (silly, incongruous, flat)
Secondary (accessory)	Delusions, hallucinations, behavioural disorder, catatonia

are manic depressive psychoses and some drug-induced states, but when using standard diagnostic criteria the diagnosis is quite reliable.

1.3 What is meant by the term 'psychosis'?

A psychosis is a severe mental illness in which the patient loses contact with reality. It is thus to be contrasted with a neurosis, for example an anxiety disorder or most forms of depression, in which people have difficulties of thinking or feeling but are, by and large, aware of their circumstances. The core features of a psychosis are symptoms such as hallucinations and delusions, which make it impossible for people to communicate clearly because their brain is literally playing tricks on them. Surrounded by false information on all sides, patients therefore often cannot make appropriate judgements on how to behave or how to respond to the world around them. The psychoses can be grouped into three major types: schizophrenia and schizophrenia-like states, manic depressive disorders and 'organic' disorders. The latter include a range of neurological and metabolic brain disorders (e.g. brain tumour and hypothyroidism) that can cause psychological symptoms, such as hallucinations, that may mimic schizophrenia.

1.4 Is schizophrenia the same as dementia praecox?

The old term 'dementia praecox' was coined by an eminent German psychiatrist, Emil Kraepelin (1856–1926), in the late 19th century. It essentially encompassed the same range of symptoms, such as hallucinations and delusions, thought disorder and a decline in social functioning. The term 'praecox' was used because it was generally seen in earlier life (i.e. the teens and 20s) and 'dementia' because it was thought to be incurable. 'Schizophrenia' came to replace it during the first half of the 20th century as a reaction to psychological and psychoanalytic insights and in an attempt to encapsulate a more positive notion of serious mental illness. Both terms were used, somewhat indiscriminately depending on the theoretical bias of the psychiatrist, until the 1950s. 'Schizophrenia' (despite its rather woolly definition) became accepted language, partly because it was a single word and partly because of the dominance of psychoanalytic theories, especially in the USA.

1.5 Is schizophrenia really a disease of modern times?

Although schizophrenia was first formally described in the 20th century, there is plentiful evidence of patients with very similar conditions in past times. The earliest description by a mental health specialist is probably that by John Haslam, apothecary to Bethlem Hospital ('Bedlam'; *Fig. 1.2*) in his *Observations on Madness and Melancholy* of 1809. The lack of medical descriptions before that has led to a theory of schizophrenia being caused by industrialization and urbanization in the 19th century. The notion even of some chronic virus has been put forward. However, depictions of very similar symptoms in medical writings, as well as in religious or dramatic literature, seem to suggest that it has always been around. For example, in Shakespeare's *King Lear* (1605), the hero has to pretend to be a typically mad 'Tom of Bedlam', and the symptoms put into his mouth are very like those of schizophrenia. It has more recently been suggested therefore that schizophrenia is part of the consequences of enhanced brain development in *Homo sapiens* and may have an evolutionary basis.

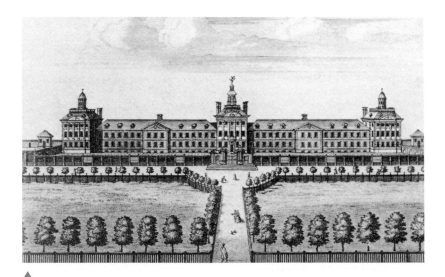

▲

Fig. 1.2 The second Bethlem, built in 1675–76. Reproduced from Scull, Andrew T 1979 Museums of Madness. Allen Lane, London

1.6   Is schizophrenia really a diagnosis, or is it just a social label?

The lack of definition of the traditional symptoms, as described by Eugen Bleuler (*see Table 1.4*), meant that the diagnosis of schizophrenia became increasingly used for a wide range of problematic patients. Anyone who was a little odd, eccentric or isolated, particularly if they were seeing a psychoanalyst in the USA, or going against the Communist Party line in the USSR, could easily be 'labelled' as suffering from schizophrenia. A clever experiment, carried out by a clinical psychologist and colleagues, showed that virtually anyone could get into hospital (private hospitals in the USA) simply by saying they heard the voice of someone saying 'thud' and claiming to be troubled by it.[2] Likewise in the USSR, the KGB conjured up a new terminology 'latent' or 'sluggish' schizophrenia, which was used to describe political dissidents and generated a considerable abuse of psychiatry in Soviet Russia.

As a result of these concerns, and a major World Health Organization study[1] showing differences in the prevalence of schizophrenia in those two countries compared with most others, a concerted effort was undertaken to adopt standardized operational definitions. These have been successful in establishing good reliability in the diagnosis of schizophrenia today, current standard classifications being *The International Classification of Diseases, ICD-10* (the tenth edition), and *The Diagnostic and Statistical Manual of Mental Disorders, DSM-IV* (the fourth edition). The former is largely a European and British arrangement and the latter American, but they are broadly similar in their descriptions of schizophrenic illnesses.

1.7   Do people who are 'paranoid' always feel persecuted?

The term 'paranoia' is generally equated with persecutory feelings or the sense that someone is harassing you or out to get you. In fact, it has a broader meaning in that paranoid individuals essentially feel in a special relationship to the world around them and tend to make the coincidental become significant. This belief system can take on grandiose or erotic forms, or even present as a morbid jealousy towards one's partner. Thus, the paranoid man may decide that the person he thinks he is being followed by is out to get him *or* is in love with him *or* worships him as a prophet. The sense of being persecuted may be the popular meaning but is not necessarily the only version of 'paranoid' in terms of patient presentation.

1.8   What is meant by the term 'catatonia'?

Catatonia is a form of relatively acute presentation of psychosis. It is characterized by abnormality of muscle tone, behavioural oddities (e.g. a repeated gesture or standing stock still for hours at a time) that can include stereotyped movements and mutism, and a tendency to adopt unusual postures. Catatonia is now uncommon, probably because of the effectiveness of modern diagnosis and the earlier use of antipsychotic medications. It reflects the physical basis of illnesses such as schizophrenia and can occur in other psychiatric and neurological conditions (*Table 1.2*). The classic presentation is that of 'waxy flexibility' whereby it is possible for patients to be put in odd, semi-rigid positions that – however uncomfortable – they maintain, just like a child's doll.

1.9 Why do people use the term 'hebephrenia'?

This word derives from the Greek goddess of youth, Hebe, and encapsulates a form of schizophrenia coming on in younger people (i.e. in their teens) with a rather characteristic pattern of symptoms. Patients tend to withdraw or decline gradually, for example in terms of school performance. They become somewhat secretive and avoidant towards their families, and develop a mixture of negative symptoms, vague hallucinations and inconsequential comments. A pattern of laughing to themselves, poor self-care and prevalent perplexity is typical. It is a form of the illness that tends to have a relatively limited or poor prognosis and very much fits the notion of 'dementia praecox' (*see Q. 1.4*).

1.10 Are there any good descriptions of schizophrenia in the historical literature?

There are numerous examples, going back to John Haslam (1810), Shakespeare (*King Lear*) and a number of medieval theses. It is also clear from the religious literature that certain of the saints had very typical symptoms of social withdrawal, while hearing voices (e.g. of God or the Holy Spirit) or developing strange beliefs about themselves. It seems highly likely that King Henry VI heard voices, which impaired his ability to rule the kingdom (and maybe influenced the resulting Wars of the Roses), and there are also snippets in classical literature. Unfortunately, there is no single good collection of these, but many of the standard histories of

---

TABLE 1.2 Some causes of catatonia

■ Schizophrenia
■ Bipolar affective disorder
■ Encephalitis
■ Carbon monoxide poisoning
■ Brain tumours
■ Heavy metal poisoning
■ Parkinsonism
■ Dementias
■ Drug-induced

psychiatry provide some references. Some brief (potential) presentations are outlined in *Table 1.3*.

1.11 Have the symptoms of schizophrenia always been the same down the years?

There seems little argument that the core symptoms, such as hallucinations, delusions and thought disorder, have been part of the established syndrome since its first description in 1911. What has changed, however, has been the *content* of patients' delusions. Thus, instead of believing that a steam engine has been placed in your head, it is now more likely that you will talk about computer chips or laser beams interfering with your thinking. It also seems true that the prevalence of catatonic schizophrenia has declined, such patients apparently being common in asylums until the 1950s. The increasing number of paranoid forms of schizophrenia (i.e. forms in which people's thoughts and perceptions, rather than strange behaviours,

---

TABLE 1.3 Schizophrenia in history

1 One believes himself to be a sparrow; a cock or an earthen vase; another a god, carrying gravely a stalk of straw and imagining himself holding a sceptre of the world' (Aretaeus of Cappadocia, *On the Causes and Signs of Diseases*, c. 150–200 AD)

2 'he indeed used but very brief speech' – tended to remain completely immobile for very long periods – 'is reported … to have often seen the Lord Jesus held in the hand … and as he lay hid an audible voice (vox corporalis) sounded in his ears for some seventeen days' (Shakespeare, *Henry VI*, 1422–1471)

3 'Poor Tom that eats the swimming frog, … that in the fury of his heart when the foul fiend rages, eats cow-dung … who is whipped from tithing to tithing … the foul fiend haunts poor Tom in the voice of a nightingale' (Shakespeare, *King Lear*, 1605)

4 'Mania and insanity are such depravations of the mind that their victims imagine, judge, and remember things falsely … doing everything unreasonable. Some … openly declare that they are possessed by a demon … and often remain mute for the longest time' (Felix Platter, 1664)

5 'Miss Hume a young lady aged 24 …, she talked extremely incoherent, so much, that she seldom finished any sentence she began, but run into some idea quite different from that she set out with, laughed and cried at times, but both without reason' (Dr John Monro's *Casebook*, 1776)

6 'Kiteing – This is a very singular and distressing mode of assailment … as boys raise a kite in the air so these wretches, by means of the air-loom and magnetic impregnations, contrive to lift into the brain some particular idea, which floats and undulates in the intellect for hours together' (John Haslam, *Illustration of Madness*, 1810)

dominate) has also been reported. This is probably due to the better recognition of such symptoms, by GPs, family and specialists. Nevertheless, comparing casebook descriptions of patients in the 19th century and patients today, one sees in general a remarkable similarity between the two.

1.12 What treatments have been given to people with schizophrenia?

The nature of the illness has led to a range of desperate remedies being tried because effective treatment for schizophrenia via medication only became available when chlorpromazine was introduced in the early 1950s (*see also Ch. 6*). Prior to that, in the 1930s and 40s, patients underwent insulin coma therapy, electroconvulsive therapy (ECT) and frontal lobotomy, with varying degrees of success. In the 1920s, there was also a vogue for 'focal infection', and numerous operations to remove appendices, colons, tonsils, etc. were carried out. There have also been various psychological approaches (*see Ch. 7*), including individual psychoanalysis, while treatment with 'monkey glands', special potions and a range of alternative nostrums has continued to this day. This variety of therapies reflects the difficulty, historically and to some extent still today, of achieving a true 'cure'.

1.13 Is ECT effective for schizophrenia?

Several controlled trials have shown that patients with paranoid schizophrenia do in fact improve after ECT. This does not mean that they do not still need antipsychotic agents, but ECT probably did some good in its heyday (the 1940s and 50s). It is not a standard treatment of schizophrenia today but is worth considering in patients with a strong affective component (i.e. mood swings) or in those in whom depression is particularly prominent. The recent National Institute for Clinical Excellence guidelines have supported this approach.

1.14 How did they treat schizophrenia before modern drugs?

The standard approach to the management of schizophrenia was placement in an asylum. A range of treatments was attempted, using 'moral' as well as physical means (*see Q. 1.12*); but this was essentially a process of removing patients from the risk of being in public and trying to care for their physical, social and behavioural needs. The rising numbers of asylum inmates, peaking in the mid-1950s, to a large degree reflected this accumulation of chronic patients. The continuing need for asylum-style care, for the 20–30% of patients who do not get better, has been a core problem for community-based approaches. The traditional principles of rehabilitation, social structure and psychosocial skills training – via specific forms of, for example, occupational therapy – have been extremely helpful in maintaining the dignity of very damaged patients. Of course, in pre-asylum times (i.e. before the early 19th century), whipping, chaining, purging and even burning at the stake (as a witch) were the likely methods of dealing with the 'furious mad'.

1.15 What is meant by the term 'hallucination'?

An hallucination is a perception in the absence of a stimulus. Thus, the patient may hear a voice, even though no one else present can hear that voice. Although auditory hallucinations (usually in the form of voices, although other sounds, such as thuds and sighs, may also be heard) are the commonest type, patients may hallucinate in any of the five sensory modalities (sight, sound, smell, taste, touch). Visual hallucinations tend to be associated with alcohol or drug dependence or forms of organic brain disorder, whereas tactile (something touching you or even biting you) and olfactory hallucinations are often missed because not enquired about. These experiences seem absolutely real to most patients, who will brook no argument that they are not actually happening.

1.16 What is understood by the term 'delusion'?

A delusion is a false belief, held with absolute conviction, despite all arguments against it. It dominates the patient's thinking and attitudes towards the world and does not accord with their sociocultural background. Delusional beliefs are often bizarre or unusual but may be as banal as being convinced that the neighbours are teasing you because they do not like the colour of your hair. Primary delusions arise de novo from the nature of the illness, whereas secondary delusions occur usually as a consequence of mood disorders (such as mania); for example, you start to believe that you are a prophet or very rich because of the aroused and manic mood that informs your pattern of thinking.

1.17 What is the difference between a delusion, an idea of reference and an illusion?

Whereas a delusion is a false belief, held with absolute conviction, an idea of reference is a sense of especial self-consciousness that someone can be argued out of. Thus, patients who worry that people are, or might be, following them can be distinguished from those convinced that the FBI *are* following them with an intent to harm. Anyone can have an idea of reference, for example when going into a room full of strangers and thinking rather self-consciously that everyone is looking at you.

By contrast an illusion is a misperception in that one mistakes a real object for something else. Thus, one may see a face in the window in the half-dark, although it may in fact be a distortion of a patterned curtain. By contrast with an hallucination, where the brain literally makes up a hologram that seems real, an illusion involves getting it wrong about something that really is there.

1.18 What is meant by the phrase 'passivity experience'?

Passivity experience is the sense that you are no longer in active control of your thoughts, feelings or movements. It can lead to people holding their arms or legs in particular positions, or doing things that they do not feel they are responsible for. It can extend to the sense that thoughts are being put into your head, or that you are being made to think or feel things about what is going on around you. It is sometimes described as having a 'loss of ego boundaries' in that individuals do not know what things are to do with them and what things are to do with the outside world. Passivity experience is one of the first-rank symptoms of schizophrenia, and such experiences are often central to a patient's hiding away from the apparent bombardment of imposed experiences.

1.19 What are the definitions of thought broadcast, thought withdrawal and thought insertion?

These encapsulate the range of delusional beliefs about thinking that characterize further aspects of the positive symptoms of schizophrenia. The term 'thought broadcast' describes a sense of other people reading your mind, in that your thoughts are exposed to public view. This sense of telepathy, or people knowing what you are thinking, can be very distressing and can lead to various unusual behaviours or forms of dress, for example wearing dark glasses or a large hat. Thought withdrawal is the sense that your thoughts are being taken away from your head or literally 'sucked out of your brain', and is usually a response to one's mind going empty and feeling that this has been caused by something else. Thought insertion is the opposite in that thoughts that do not seem to be one's own appear in one's mind. They therefore seem to be alien in some way, so one feels that someone else has put them into one's head. This may be attributed to some form of malign purpose, a computer program, a laser beam or some other form of special experience. Patients usually describe only one or two of all these states, rather than having them all at any one time (*Fig. 1.3*).

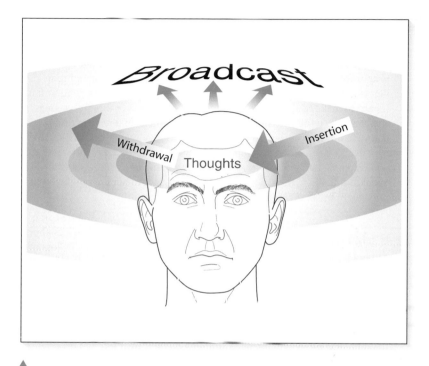

Fig. 1.3 Pictorial representation of thought broadcast, thought withdrawal, and thought insertion. Note that patients generally experience only one or two of these phenomena, not a 'full house'.

1.20 What's a positive symptom and what's a negative symptom?

By and large, schizophrenic symptoms are grouped as being either positive or negative, in that the former are additions to one's normal pattern of thinking or feeling, whereas the latter are deficits (*see Tables 2.1 and 2.2, Box 2.1, Q. 2.6, Q. 2.10–2.12 and Q. 2.23*). The typical positive symptoms are delusions and hallucinations, so characteristic of severe mental illness, as well as formal thought disorder (e.g. thought broadcast and thought block) and passivity experience. The negative symptoms include loss of drive, a flattened affect (i.e. being fatuous or incongruous), social withdrawal, difficulty in thinking and self-neglect. A poorer prognosis is generally associated with negative symptoms, especially if there is an associated cognitive impairment.

1.21   What does 'schizoid' mean?

'Schizoid' is a term outlining a particular form of personality style. It does not necessarily precede the onset of a schizophrenic illness, although a proportion of people with schizoid characters do develop schizophrenic illnesses. The term describes individuals who tend to be loners, tend to find it hard to make relationships, tend to dwell on their own internal feelings and thoughts more persistently than those of others, and tend to find it hard to communicate with other people. The term 'schizotypal personality disorder' in particular stresses an appearance of aloofness, eccentric habits, poor rapport, rather vague or stereotyped thinking and even what is termed 'magical thinking'. There does seem to be a greater incidence of schizotypal disorder in the families of patients with schizophrenia.

1.22   Is schizophrenia just grown-up autism?

Although there are some similar symptoms, infantile autism seems by and large to be an entirely separate disorder from schizophrenia. There is no relationship whatsoever between having autism in childhood and developing schizophrenia, and there is no evidence, for example, that autistic patients experience hallucinations or delusions. The term 'autism' was originally used in the description of schizophrenia (*see Table 1.1*), largely to emphasize patients' tendencies to dwell on their own internal experiences rather than communicate with the outside world. This usage must be differentiated from the formal diagnostic category of childhood autism (F84.0 in the *ICD-10*), which is the most well known of a group of conditions categorized as pervasive developmental disorders. Furthermore, childhood autism comes on before the age of 3, whereas schizophrenia is usually an illness of late adolescence or the early 20s.

1.23   Is schizophrenia what used to be called hysteria or neurasthenia?

No. Whereas it is likely that a number of patients labelled 'hysterical' in the 19th century might have had schizophrenic symptoms as well, there is no evidence that the over-dramatization of symptoms, or having psychosomatic symptoms with no organic basis, is associated with schizophrenic patients. Likewise, the term 'neurasthenia' describes a sense of being tired all the time and feeling depressed and anxious, and it is probably now likely to present as a depressive illness rather than schizophrenia. There have probably been a number of terms used to describe patients with schizophrenia in the past, and one would need to look at the actual symptoms outlined in order to clarify what really was the matter with them.

1. 24 Are most murderers psychotic or schizophrenic?

No. The proportion of homicides committed by patients with schizophrenia has been declining consistently over the past 40 years. This may be an artefact of the figures or a function of the rising tide of violence in urban society. Suffice it to say that only about 20 murders a year in the UK (among the 500–600 that take place) can be attributed to psychotic patients. The attribution of criminality or enhanced risk to patients with schizophrenia has been one of the most damaging aspects of modern community care, leading to the rise of 'risk management', the enhancement of stigma and social isolation for a number of patients. Even when patients with schizophrenia are associated with homicides, there are commonly other factors, such as a personality disorder and/or drug or alcohol dependence, that compound the picture. Patients with schizophrenia are much more likely to be the victims than the perpetrators of violence, abuse and exploitation.

1. 25 What is 'simple' schizophrenia?

This is an uncommon type of schizophrenia in which there is apparently no evidence of delusions, hallucinations or other obviously psychotic features. Patients simply seem to evolve into being more withdrawn, odd and self-absorbed, even becoming aimless and idle, just like those with 'negative symptoms'. It can be difficult to distinguish this as a real illness separate from the solitary, perhaps eccentric, behaviour of those with a 'schizoid' temperament. Some researchers consider this to be a non-viable category, whereas others view it as the later stages of an illness in which the more florid symptoms have passed unnoticed by the family or been covered up by the patient. *Table 1.4* provides an outline of traditional categories and their symptoms.

1.26 Do paranoia and schizophrenia always go together?

Not necessarily. Although paranoid schizophrenia seems to be the commonest type diagnosed today, it has always been understood that a

TABLE 1.4 Symptoms of the traditional forms of schizophrenia

	Hallucinations	Delusions	Thought disorder	Passivity	Behavioural abnormalities	Negative
Paranoid	++	++	+	+	+/−	−
Hebephrenic	+	?	++	+	+	+
Catatonic	+	?	?	+	+++	−
Simple	−	−	−	−	−	+++

?, not apparent but may be reported after recovery

number of individuals simply develop a paranoid belief, or set of beliefs, without any of the other symptoms, such as hallucinations or thought disorder, that accompany schizophrenia. These patients were historically (*see Fig. 1.1*) considered to have a 'pure' form of paranoia, but this is now termed 'delusional disorder'. Many schizophrenic patients, therefore, are certainly not paranoid, coming across instead as perhaps timid, silly or even slightly buffoon-like. It is important to distinguish these two conditions, not least because many people are misdiagnosed because they seem to develop paranoid reactions to drugs (e.g. cannabis and amphetamines) or in association with excessive alcohol intake (*see also Q 2.19*).

1.27 Do schizophrenic patients have reduced sexual activity and fertility?

This used to be the standard teaching, not least because schizophrenic patients, especially male patients who become ill earlier, tend to remain unmarried. Furthermore, since, until the 1970s, patients largely lived in asylums, they clearly had a much more limited ability to beget children. Yet the prevalence of schizophrenia seems remarkably consistent over time and across countries, and there is no evidence that the illness in itself impairs sexual function. Many patients in fact develop enduring and strangely affectionate relationships, often with other sufferers, and with current community care policies most clinicians now mainly concern themselves with the effects of antipsychotic drugs on sexual activity. There was even a 19th-century theory that excessive masturbation caused insanity, which probably derived from physicians actually witnessing patients doing this in those large impersonal asylums. These theories of infertility and masturbation very much reflect the speculations and ignorance that have surrounded this condition down the years.

1.28 What is meant by the term 'pseudohallucination'?

This essentially means the experience of having a hallucination – for example hearing a voice – that one knows is not real. That is to say, patients will describe a voice, or at least a voice-like experience, telling them to do things, which takes place inside their head. Unlike the 'true' hallucinations associated with schizophrenia, the voice does not seem to come from another person, for example, or to comment about the patient in the third person. Furthermore, the experience will seem to be part of one's own mental make-up rather than, for example, being *imposed* from outside, and patients also seem to have some control in terms of putting it out of their minds. It is sometimes quite difficult to distinguish this experience from true hallucinations, but it can be important in distinguishing drug-induced states and forms of personality disorder, from true schizophrenia. Of course, pseudohallucinations do not necessarily exclude schizophrenia, and distinguishing between presentations usually requires considerable experience.

1.29 Is schizophrenia really an illness, in the sense of diabetes or arthritis?

There seems no doubt that schizophrenia is just as much a physical illness as are a range of common conditions such as diabetes, multiple sclerosis and psoriasis. Chronicity is an established feature with all of these, our current treatments being based on maintaining remission. Of course, the pathological basis of schizophrenia remains an enigma, but there is sufficient evidence for most psychiatrists now to see it as a subtle form of brain disease with primarily psychological symptoms. There are some clues to its physical basis in terms of ventricular enlargement on brain scans, catatonic symptoms such as waxy flexibility, and the unusual physical presentations associated with high physiological arousal (e.g. clothing inappropriate for the ambient temperature).

Neuropathological studies likewise have consistently shown smaller neurons, especially in the hippocampus and pre-frontal cortex, which have less complex structures in terms of axons and dendrites. Thus, the nervous 'wiring' is different, not connecting up as intricately, with a state of so-called 'dysconnectivity'. Furthermore, symptoms such as thought disorder and hallucinations are just what one would expect of abnormalities in those parts of the brain which organize perception and cognition.

PQ PATIENT QUESTIONS

1.30 If I've got schizophrenia, does it mean I've gone mad?

Although suffering from schizophrenia means that patients may have some unusual experiences, for example hearing voices, it does not necessarily mean that they are not aware of or sensible to this. Schizophrenia can certainly be very disabling, making it hard to think or concentrate, and making one's family very anxious. However, people working with those suffering from schizophrenia often consider such patients to be remarkably honest, to have a good sense of right and wrong, and to cope quite phlegmatically with some very distressing symptoms.

If there is any meaning at all to the word 'mad', it is that people do not comply with the accepted customs or behaviours of their society. Anyone can be called mad – and it is a very widely used word – if they just do something a bit out of the ordinary. This could be getting drunk, stripping naked and jumping into an icy pond, as many people do on New Year's Day for example, or simply getting in a muddle and taking the wrong train. The important thing to understand is that doing something slightly out of the ordinary, although it may be the result of a mental illness such as schizophrenia, is more often than not just a personal eccentricity.

It is also important to realize that many people do recover from schizophrenia, that it is a real illness, and that some of the symptoms are not very different from normal human experiences, albeit writ large. For example, anyone can hallucinate if very tired or disorientated, and nearly 30% of people report hearing a voice or odd sounds, sometimes, for example when drifting in or out of sleep (so-called 'hypnagogic' or 'hypnopompic' hallucinations).

1.31 Have there been many changes or advances in treating schizophrenia over the past century?

Yes. As outlined in *Table 1.5* (*see also Q. 1.12*), much has happened, especially over the past 50 years. From having just to put people in asylums in order to keep them fed, watered, occupied (possibly) and out of harm's way, it has become more and more possible to treat them effectively and give them something of a normal life. The use of drug treatments, changes in mental health legislation and new social and psychological approaches have all played their part. The severity of the illness has been reduced, more than two-thirds of patients now being out of hospital – compared with once over 90% being 'asylum inmates' – and there has been a major expansion of resources in terms of nurses, social workers and psychiatrists.

TABLE 1.5 Modern advances in the management and treatment of schizophrenia

1952	Chlorpromazine – the first effective 'neuroleptic' – introduced in France
1950s and 60s	Haloperidol (1958 in Belgium) and numerous other typical antipsychotics introduced
1956	Peak of asylum inpatient figures, which fall steadily thereafter as community care develops
1959	New Mental Health Act, allowing voluntary admission and abolishing 'certification' via the courts
1970s	Clozapine introduced but withdrawn (because of agranulocytosis); reintroduced 1990
	Depot injections introduced
	Diagnostic improvements via World Health Organization studies
1980s	Family psycho-educational and cognitive therapies
1983	Mental Health Act – improved patient rights/tribunals
1990s	Atypical agents introduced – risperidone (1993), olanzapine (1996), quetiapine and amisulpride (1997), zotepine (1998)
1999	National Service Framework for Mental Health
2002	National Institute of Clinical Excellence guidelines for schizophrenia management (www.nice.org.uk)

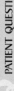
PQ PATIENT QUESTIONS

Symptoms of schizophrenia

2

2.1   What is the commonest symptom of schizophrenia?

The symptom most commonly reported in all major surveys is that of experiencing auditory hallucinations. These will occur in approximately 70–80% of patients at some time in the course of their illness. Psychiatrists try to distinguish between third-person auditory hallucinations – that is to say voices talking about 'him' or 'her' – rather than second-person hallucinations, in which the voices talk to 'you'. Thus, auditory hallucinations diagnostic of a true schizophrenic illness will consist of hearing conversations going on about oneself, for example 'Look what he's doing; he seems to be walking rather fast', and patients will often recognize a particular voice by a given name or personality. The experience is of course entirely real to the sufferer (like a radio being switched on nearby). Patients sometimes give such a convincing description or explanation that the examining doctor does not realize that auditory hallucinations are being described (*see also* Q. 3.2).

2.2   Does schizophrenia really have clear and defined symptoms?

By and large it does, and there is considerable reliability in the diagnosis even among psychiatrists from different cultures or with different primary languages. Agreement approaches some 80–90% in those appropriately trained. The basis of this reliability has been a considerable research effort by the World Health Organization, a constant refining of research diagnostic criteria and the extensive use of Schneider's first-rank symptoms (*Table 2.1*). The main difficulties occur in the early stages of the illness and in the fact that one sometimes has to work very hard at extracting definite symptoms from embarrassed, frightened or semi-mute patients. Good-quality history-taking, including a corroborative history from another individual, as well as very careful and ongoing examinations of mental state, are thus core features of modern psychiatry.

2.3   Are there any specific physical signs or biochemical abnormalities that are indicative of a schizophrenic illness?

The simple answer is no. Physical examination is, almost by definition, always normal unless the illness is secondary to, for example, a form of encephalitis or the patient happens to have an associated condition (e.g. diabetes). Some patients show 'soft signs' of mild neurological impairment in terms of coordination, elicited, for example, by getting them to tap out patterns on a piece of paper in a regular rhythm or to supinate/pronate their wrists together and/or in sequence.

Likewise, there are no established haematological, biochemical or radiological abnormalities, although routine blood tests are carried out on first admission as part of the elimination of other potential causative or

---

TABLE 2.1 Schneider's first-rank symptoms

'Wherever such experiences [first-rank symptoms] can be established with certainty, and no underlying physical illness can be found, we speak clinically in all modesty of schizophrenia' (Kurt Schneider, *Clinical Psychopathology*, 1959, trans. M.W. Hamilton)

Auditory hallucinations	As a running commentary on one's actions As a voice repeating one's own thoughts (also known as *écho de la pensée*) In the third person, calling the patient 'he' or 'she'
Formation of delusions	As a delusional perception whereby a normal perception (e.g. seeing a light turn green) leads directly to a fully formed delusion (e.g. believing you are the angel Gabriel)
Passivity experience	Thoughts, feelings or actions are experienced as being controlled by other people or agencies, making one the *passive* recipient rather than the active initiator
Thought insertion/ broadcast/withdrawal	Experiencing one's thoughts as being put into or taken out of one's head, and/or being known about by (broadcast to) other people

NB Individual symptoms often overlap to some degree, for example patients' feeling that voices control them *and* interfere with their thoughts. Each first-rank symptom should be seen as just one possible ingredient in an often complex pattern of experience.

---

associated conditions. There have been a number of false dawns in this respect, one of the most recent in the UK being the apparent finding of a 'pink spot' in the urine, which was subsequently discredited. Increasingly sophisticated research techniques, for example in radio isotope scanning, are beginning to pick up some abnormalities in individual patients, but we still do not have any kind of definitive diagnostic test for schizophrenia.

2.4 Do patients with schizophrenia have any typical physical abnormalities?

No. Again, there has been a rich history of attempts at diagnosis based on body shape (e.g. 'pyknic') or size, or head shape or size (dolicocephaly), but these have all proved entirely unreliable. If patients are suffering from catatonia, they may demonstrate waxy flexibility, but this is rare. Likewise, from the behavioural point of view, many patients seem to dress inappropriately, for example wearing layers of clothing in hot weather or walking around with their shirt undone in the freezing cold. These are indicative and interesting rather than diagnostic.

2.5 What is the best way of establishing whether someone really is 'hearing voices' (i.e. experiencing auditory hallucinations)?

Questioning

Since there is no unequivocal scientific test, this must be carried out via direct examination and questioning, specialist observation or clarifying the history from friends or relatives. Unless patients directly come out with the complaint, for example that people seem to be talking about them or harassing them, or even 'calling me dirty names in the street', the doctor has to be prepared to ask 'Have you had any unusual experiences' or 'Are the neighbours bothering you?' The blunt question 'Do you hear voices?' may be appropriate for patients with chronic illness, whose symptoms are being evaluated in the course of ongoing treatment, but rarely gets much response in the troubled, first-onset, withdrawn young psychotic who considers his experiences real and thus genuinely does not think he is hearing voices. Such intrusive questions should also be saved up for the latter part of an interview when some rapport and trust will hopefully have been established. Introducing the question with phrases such as 'It's not uncommon when people have been troubled or upset that strange things happen…' or 'It sometimes seems like our minds are literally talking to us; has that ever happened to you?' can sometimes get a more informative reply.

Observation

If, despite reasonably detailed, and perhaps repeated, mental state examinations, nothing seems to emerge, direct observation at home or in hospital can be very useful. Mothers will report hearing their sons talking to themselves or crying out in their rooms at night, while the whole purpose of an inpatient admission is to use the skills of the nursing staff. This will involve observing behaviours, seeing how patients become distracted or start talking at objects or walls, and listening to patients seeming to have conversations with others in their rooms. Depending on the cultural background, regular praying and chanting or playing loud music (sometimes with headphones on), in order to drown out 'the voices', can also be indirect signs of hallucinatory experiences.

Social behaviour

For individuals living alone, this all becomes much more difficult. Discussions with the neighbours can sometimes be enlightening since they may also have complained to the police or housing authorities about unusual shouting, calling out or other loud noises next door (*Case vignette 2.1*). Secondary behaviours generated by constantly 'hearing voices' include bombarding noise nuisance lines, banging on the ceiling or walls (the little round indentations of a broom handle are almost diagnostic) and constantly moving from place to place because of feeling threatened or harassed (by voices, etc.). Constant complaints to the housing, gas or electricity authorities may also reflect reactions to psychotic experiences.

CASE VIGNETTE 2.1

A 35-year-old man was transferred from hospital to a flat in his local East London community. He had been treated for a fairly severe schizophrenic illness with regular medication while in hospital, and his symptoms had responded well. Because of side-effects, he had been changed from a depot to an oral medication 3 months before discharge, but he remained stable in terms of his mental state. He preferred to live alone, and a social worker from a community mental health team was assigned to support him and see him regularly.

Over the next few months he seemed to have remained quite stable at home. He dressed properly, looked after his flat and regularly attended a day centre. Although the social worker was relatively inexperienced, she felt that he was quite amenable in his presentation and seemed to be keeping up a good appearance. He did, however, miss an outpatient appointment with his psychiatrist, apologizing for forgetting, but then missed another one 4 weeks later.

One of the neighbours became increasingly concerned about the noise at night and talked to her landlord. The police were informed, as were the housing authorities, but nothing further happened because all seemed well during an evening visit by the social worker and a colleague.

The neighbours, however, became more and more concerned and contacted social services; a further assessment was therefore arranged at home. Again, the patient was friendly, denied any symptoms and agreed to go and see a psychiatrist. Before this appointment was reached, he unfortunately had an argument with another patient at the day centre and stabbed him. Arrested and assessed in custody, it became clear, after proper examination, that the man had in fact been hearing unpleasant, derogatory hallucinations for quite a while and was attributing this to people at his day centre, which led to his untoward behaviour. A better understanding of auditory hallucinations, by all those involved, and a quicker examination and assessment by an experienced doctor, could well have prevented this outcome.

2.6 What is meant by the term 'thought disorder'?

In technical terms, this describes the disruption of one's normal pattern of thoughts, which should generally be expressed in coherent language. Speech becomes rather diffuse and rambling, patients trailing off in mid-sentence and using language in a rather idiosyncratic way. They may make up new phrases or new words (neologisms) or give an established word (or phrase) a personal meaning (metonym). Other terms used to describe this include 'derailment', the image being of the train of thought literally going off the tracks, and 'knight's move thinking', reflecting the curious move allowed to the knight on a chessboard.

It is sometimes so difficult to follow what a patient is saying that the term 'word salad' is appropriate in that there seems to be just a jumble of words and phrases, tossed around as in a salad bowl, with little obvious connection between them. At other times, examining physicians feel that they are somehow getting out of their depth as the patient goes into a complex explanation of implants, toxic chemicals or some other topic. This personal reaction, of not being able to understand what the patient is saying or of finding it hard to concentrate on what is being said is often a rather good diagnostic pointer. Experienced psychiatrists can pick up very quickly why they cannot follow someone's train of thought, but those not used to dealing with thought disorder may worry that it is their own limitations of knowledge or comprehension. This perplexity – which often turns to exasperation – can be seen as reflecting the patient's own incoherence. Some examples of thought disorder are outlined in *Box 2.1*.

2.7 Do patients with schizophrenia often show forms of movement disorder?

 Untreated patients, particularly if they come into the category of catatonic schizophrenia, often show abnormal movements. These include unusual postures maintained for a long period of time, the 'waxy flexibility' whereby a patient can be literally placed like a piece of plasticine into a given position, and stereotypies, in which patients regularly repeat movements, for example waving their arms around in a regular pattern or mimicking behaviours such as saluting or marching. They may also indulge in echopraxia, that is, the automatic copying of someone else's movements, particularly those of the doctor who is interviewing them (*Box 2.2*)!

Part and parcel of some of the more chronic illnesses are the facial movements of oral dyskinesia (chewing, grimacing, schnauzkrampf – making a snout-like appearance with one's nose and mouth), although nowadays these usually arise secondary to antipsychotic medication (and are attributed thereto; *see Ch. 6*). Nevertheless, about a third of patients in Victorian asylums seem to have had some kind of movement or muscle tone disorder.

A number of forms of movement disorder, for example tremors, Parkinsonism, akathisia and tardive dyskinesia, are deemed to be side-effects of dopamine-blocking medication (*see Ch. 6*).

BOX 2.1 Examples of thought disorder

- Metonym. John Haslam's patient in *Illustrations of Madness* (1809) used the term 'lobster-cracking', by which he meant 'an external pressure of the magnetic atmosphere surrounding him, so as to stagnate his circulation, impede his vital motions and produce instant death'. Another example is the use of the word 'greenbacking' by a patient convinced that a presence was coming up behind him and putting things into his body or mind
- Neologism. This is an example from a standard textbook: 'Cordron. A theme of curved and fancy lines, … from the point on the top of the post-collic (unexplainable) word matching the point; caller from the Cordron & Crosby'. Other terms fitting this category include 'thinglement', being 'castelized' (?spelling) and being 'burbelated'. New words are of course part and parcel of living language anyway, and there is often a sense that words created by patients are somehow understandable in the context of their particular perspective
- Formal thought disorder.
  (1) This is a letter quoted in a 1927 textbook (*Textbook of Psychiatry* by D.K. Henderson and R.D. Gillespie, Oxford University Press):
  'Dear Sir, I have just had dinner. I ate my dinner, the monkey and I feel better. change I. Nurse is always making the tea. Betsy's nurse.
  Wearing for a cup of
  Tea.
  Bathing patient (Ogalvie)
  Your –
  I J G U
  Gins Druce yours sincerely,
  P.R.
  (2) A modern interview

Dr:	Tell me more about that.
Patient:	What?
Dr:	How is your usual mood?
Patient:	[laughing and then coughing] I feel like giggling, no, but I'm

  always feeling like this all my life I've been like this.

Dr:	Like what?
Patient:	Uh? Well, change every five minutes
Dr:	I see
Patient:	I can change in the middle of a sentence
Dr:	In what way?
Patient:	Well just go on to something else, it's not until two days later…

  I have told them about that, you know what I mean, I know it sometimes, I go on, and I'm saying something about something and I know

BOX 2.1 **Examples of thought disorder—cont'd**

I've and I've gone to something else and then when I'm leaving I say good God what did I [laughs] I finished what I was going to say. But I've always been like that.

And one a house looked ever so … I didn't like the top or the bottom one I was doing two, and I had a point like that, while I walked and I had my bag with me then, I took too much baggage you know, I only took about six shirts, and that but it was too heavy, I took too much, you know it's amazing and you only got a little you know it ain't too much … six rows of…

BOX 2.2 **Physical/behavioural signs in schizophrenia***

- Ill-fitting or unusual clothes
- Heavily nicotine-stained fingers
- Slightly uncoordinated gait
- Odd grimacing, e.g. schnauzkrampf
- Impaired coordination on motor tasks
- Physiological arousal (although blood pressure and pulse are normal)

* These are only indicative and not diagnostic

2.8 Do patients with schizophrenia also have depressive symptoms?

It is not uncommon for the early stages of a schizophrenic illness to be marked by what looks like depression. Patients withdraw or stop eating, seem sad and unhappy, and describe being 'depressed', and a number clearly do have associated, true depressive symptoms. Claims of feeling 'depressed' should always be closely examined because this will often be occurring secondary to the unpleasant experiences patients are experiencing, for example abusive hallucinations or the feeling that their thoughts are being interfered with or controlled. In this sense, depression can be seen as an understandable reaction to the psychotic symptoms of schizophrenia. Many patients also have sufficient insight to realize they are literally 'going mad' and simply do not want that to be true.

The treatment of schizophrenia can likewise have its depressive consequences. If it is ineffective, patients can feel hopeless and unhelped, hence the high rate of suicide (10–15% depending on one's database) in schizophrenic patients. If treatment is successful, the dawning insight into what has happened to oneself, the impairment of one's social relationships, the associated stigma and the somewhat flattening or sedating nature of some of the medications one is required to take will all combine to create a depressive picture. The potential for depression, in the context of a schizophrenic illness, is, however, a better prognostic sign than the silliness and fatuity associated with poor insight and a more deteriorated personality.

2.9 Are panic attacks common in schizophrenia?

Typical panic attacks, namely the sudden onset of an intense sense of fear, the associated physiological symptoms (palpitations, dyspnoea, chest pain, sweats, tremors, 'jelly legs') are not part of the standard symptomatology of schizophrenia. Many panicky patients do, however, describe a sense of paranoia, by which they mean enhanced self-consciousness when in public places because of their own inner states of anxiety. This is a typical symptom of agoraphobia. Distinguishing this state from the true paranoid feelings of schizophrenia is most important clinically and is one of the commonest reasons for misdiagnosis (of schizophrenia when it does not exist).

It should also be understood that patients with schizophrenia are often psychologically aroused and are very sensitive to the world around them. There is some evidence that untoward life events (e.g. threats or losses) can precipitate an enhancement of their symptoms. It is also clear that living in an atmosphere of 'high expressed emotion' (one in which they feel constantly criticized or talked about by family members who are themselves anxious) can significantly increase the chance of a relapse (*see Box 7.1*).

2.10 Why do patients with schizophrenia complain of things being done to them or of their being interfered with?

Because the nature of schizophrenic symptoms is such that they seem absolutely real, and since by definition people do not have any insight into these experiences, it is perfectly reasonable for them to complain about what is happening. The common complaints are of harassment, for example neighbours shouting at them or banging on the wall, of bullying or teasing (e.g. at school), of things being stolen from them, or of their bodies being actually interfered with. These reflect the tendency to attribute changes to something specific (i.e. making the coincidental significant), or the presence of tactile or olfactory hallucinations (i.e. feeling they are being touched or smelling unpleasant odours), which are deemed to be imposed upon them. Modern forms, for example, of 'passivity experience' can include a sense of someone interfering with them, the television giving them special personal messages or some kind of ray or poison being injected into them. Patients may even demand special X-rays or even a brain scan so that they can demonstrate their experience of what is inside them.

2.11 Are olfactory or visual hallucinations typical of schizophrenia?

See *Table 2.11* for a summary of typical types of hallucination. Whereas some 70–80% of patients experience auditory hallucinations, the prevalence of other forms of hallucination is much lower. The usual figures quoted report that between 10–20% of patients experience visual hallucinations, whereas a lesser proportion (perhaps 10%) experience olfactory hallucinations (i.e. hallucinations of smell). It may be that these are actually more common but by their very nature are less complained about because they are not so intrusive. It is not uncommon, for example, for patients to refuse food because it 'smells bad', but this may be mixed in with a sense that they are possibly being poisoned because they feel somehow changed. A classic complaint, from patients or even their relatives, is that their drink has been 'spiked' or 'drugged', thus producing their current state of mind.

Visual hallucinations must be carefully distinguished from other causes of brain disorder, complex visual hallucinations (e.g. whole scenes of people dressed in extraordinary costumes) usually being associated with quite definite cerebral pathologies.

TABLE 2.2 Types of hallucination	
Auditory	Usually 'voices' but may be just indistinct sounds. Can be abusive, friendly, nondescript, conversational or commanding
Visual	Uncommon in schizophrenia; usually small objects and not very complex in composition (much more typical in alcohol or drug withdrawal states or in association with brain disorder, e.g. tumours, epilepsy, severe migraine)
Tactile/somatic (touch)	Experience of being touched, stroked or even bitten or pinched. Includes feelings of something inside one's body (e.g. a snake or implant)
Olfactory (smell)	Unusual but well recognized. Various smells or hypersensitivity to smell – ?a miasma, classically associated with temporal lobe epilepsy and temporal lobe (especially hippocampal) tumours
Gustatory (taste)	Uncommon and may be difficult to distinguish from olfactory sensations – food tastes 'funny' or even perhaps 'poisoned'

2.12 Is it common for patients to feel they are being 'touched up' or their bodies are being changed in some way?

The types of hallucination termed 'somatic' or 'tactile' are very poorly explored in many patients' histories. It is absolutely standard for patients to feel that their bodies are being changed, some even spending hours staring in the mirror at their faces, trying to recognize themselves, and/or complaining of hair loss or a distorted nose. Some of these patients have what is called a 'pure dysmorphophobia', that is, a single delusional conviction that some part of their body (e.g. their nose) has been changed. A resort to plastic surgery is a typical concomitant of this (*see also Table 3.7*).

Other patients may decide that they have been transformed in some way, with fragments of a computer in them, or their bodies being turned to glass or concrete, and their actions will be related to that. They may even sense that their arms or legs have been detached, or that blood or fluid is pouring out of them, and they will take action (e.g. numerous bandages wrapped around their arms or legs) to stop this. Complaints of being bitten, scratched, stroked or sexually interfered with are very common and may lead to unnecessary investigations or even formal inquiries.

2.13 What if you can't understand what a patient is talking about?

As outlined in the section on thought disorder (*see Q. 2.6*), a patient's incomprehensibility is in itself often diagnostic. Part of routine psychiatric training requires a close analysis of the trains of thought of patients' language, and with continued experience it soon becomes clear what is abnormal and what is not. Doctors with less clinical experience, especially medical students, may feel that it is they themselves who are inadequate in terms of concentration, understanding or even intellect. Generally, if you cannot understand what the patient is talking about, that in itself is a definition of a form of thought disorder. Writing down just what the patient is saying, or even better getting them to talk on a dictaphone, can be very helpful in clarifying this. Once the words are typed up on a written page, it soon becomes clear how extensive and detailed some patients' thought disorders can be.

2.14 Do patients tend to make up new words or phrases or use certain terms idiosyncratically?

Diagnostic features of schizophrenia include the ability to make up new words (neologisms) and the tendency to use certain phrases or words in a highly personal, idiosyncratic way (metonyms). Detailed examples are outlined in *Q. 2.6*. The term 'portmanteau' has also been used to describe this tendency as patients tend to carry round with them a word, a phrase or several words or phrases that are idiosyncratic in describing how they feel and what their psychotic experiences are. This oddness or repetitiveness of language is a very useful diagnostic feature.

2.15 Is a belief in telepathy or mind-reading diagnostic of schizophrenia?

Not in itself. Although telepathy and mind-reading clearly derive from the typical schizophrenic experiences of thought broadcasting and thought insertion, a number of individuals nevertheless do believe in this process, hence the increased levels of research into parapsychology. It is important to distinguish whether or not patients have actually experienced these phenomena or merely believe in them because they are somewhat gullible to the more alluring articles, books or television programmes about parapsychological experiences. It may also be that certain individuals do simply have one, single, schizophrenia-like symptom (e.g. a sense of thought broadcast) without any other impairments or difficulties. In this sense, schizophrenia must be seen as a spectrum of disorder, including symptoms that can occasionally occur (if one is very tired or has taken odd drugs, for example) in otherwise 'normal' people.

2.16 Is it typical for patients with schizophrenia to lose touch with their friends?

Unfortunately, yes. This can occur in a variety of ways. The illness itself is most stigmatizing, and patients often withdraw from social contact, act oddly in public places or will embarrass their friends by their statements. Once hospitalized, they will have lost contact with their peer group and fall behind in terms of school, college or work. Because of the effects of medication, the difficulty in motivating themselves and the (not uncommon) problems with concentration that are part and parcel of the illness, schizophrenia sufferers find it hard to maintain a job, converse easily with others or acquire new skills. Applying for jobs is daunting, and illness declarations necessary for occupational health purposes create the double-bind of covering up (and thus falsifying information) or quickly being rejected because of the stigma.

2.17 Is talking to yourself a typical sign of schizophrenia?

Yes and no. Yes, in the sense that one of the most obvious signs to spot when a patient is suffering from auditory hallucinations is the tendency, not unnatural in most of us, to answer back. Patients will describe this in varying ways. Some will say they are having a dialogue with what seems to be a genuine person talking to them. Others will answer back in order to try and drown the voices out or even shut them up. Some patients seem to describe hallucinations, yet if one looks at them closely it is as if the hallucinations derive from their own larynx (which seems to be moving in a voice-like way). The crude behavioural observation, from families, neighbours or nurses, that individuals are constantly talking to themselves, for example in the privacy of their own rooms, usually means that hallucinations are part of the picture.

However, many people talk to themselves, as a personal idiosyncrasy, because of loneliness or just out of habit. The act of talking to oneself is of itself *not* diagnostic and should never be seen as such. It is at most an indicator, guiding one to a further assessment. The typical figure of the tramp walking along the street muttering to himself may therefore reflect chronic schizophrenia, a drug/alcohol-induced state or a degree of brain damage. Now that mobile phones are ubiquitous (one patient campaigner even suggesting that a mobile phone would be a useful disguise for those with the talking-to-themselves tendency), this is not so uncommon a sight on the average city street. Like all common platitudes, it has a core of truth that needs to be put into context.

2.18 Is there anything about the way people dress themselves or do their hair that is typical of schizophrenia (*see also Box 2.2*)?

Most people with schizophrenia are relatively indistinguishable from the way they dress or groom. The main impact of their illness, in this sense, is poverty and the likelihood therefore of poorly fitting, non-designer clothes. However, eccentric clothing, not uncommonly a touch colourful and not quite hanging together, is quite common in some patients. This may reflect their genuine inability to interpret the meaning of appearances (e.g. understand people's facial expressions) or may reflect a slight clumsiness that some patients have as part of their neuropsychiatric disability. Nowadays, however, the range of hairstyles deemed acceptable has become something of a help. Excessively long or strangely cut hair no longer seems anomalous, although hair abnormalities are not really even a feature indicative of a diagnosis. The tendency to pluck one's hair out regularly (trichotillomania) is a separate condition, rarely associated with schizophrenia.

2.19 Do patients with schizophrenia commonly describe suicidal feelings?

The rate of suicide among patients with schizophrenia is approximately 10–15%. Particularly in the earlier stages of the illness, when there seems to be an associated depression, be it reactive or true, patients describe feeling low, suicidal and rather frightened of some of their symptoms. Unfortunately, a number simply struggle on and cover up, the first the clinician hears of them being at a suicide inquest. The difficulty in communicating the nature of their experiences, as well as the stigma of the illness ('going mad') are probably the key factors in suicidal feelings (and acts) not being dealt with earlier.

It is important to distinguish these troubling experiences from the common casualty presentation of patients with a personality disorder, alcohol or drug problem, who are in some degree of social distress, agitatedly claiming that voices are telling them to kill themselves and that they must be admitted or they will do so. Such presentations mostly involve pseudo-hallucinations (i.e. voices from within one's head, into which one has insight, knowing they are not 'real', and which one can turn on and off by an act of will), and they will not be linked to any of the other symptoms typical of schizophrenia (*see Q 1.28*).

2.20 Is it typical of schizophrenia for someone to go mute or semi-mute?

There are not many causes for elective mutism, but it is certainly a symptom typical of the catatonic type of schizophrenia. Some patients of course simply do not want to speak, and there is actually nothing wrong with them. However, the features of psychotic mutism usually include evidence of high physiological arousal (e.g. shaking, sweating, increased pulse rate), an obviously alert facial expression, occasional attempts to articulate something and associated postures or movements that may be repetitive. Patients sometimes whisper an occasional word under their breath, for example to a parent, indicating that they do have the power of speech if necessary, whereas others can even be stuporous.

This symptom is most difficult to assess in children or adolescent patients, where the act may be much more deliberate as part of rebellion, fear or genuinely not knowing what to say or how to say it.

2.21 Do people with schizophrenia usually know that something is wrong?

By definition, schizophrenia is the kind of illness in which most (70% or more) patients do not have full insight into what is happening to them. The essence of psychotic symptoms such as hallucinations is that they are absolutely real to the sufferer. Attempts at arguing against them, certainly in the early stages, can be completely frustrating, hence the difficulties experienced by many families and/or carers. A number of patients are, however, aware that they are changing, are perplexed and 'depressed' by this and do seek help. This may well be for some kind of physical investigation (to show up the computer chip implanted into their brain) or via a request for something to deal with their anxiety or depression. Nevertheless, up to 20% of patients with schizophrenia do not actually get diagnosed, and it is not difficult for patients to slip through the net of diagnostic clarifications, especially in the early stages of not too severe illness.

2.22 What is the best way of getting someone to talk about their 'delusions'?

There is no best way to get patients to talk, but they will say – particularly when they have had delusional and/or hallucinatory experiences for quite a while – that their concerns in this area have often not been addressed. Part of the definition of a delusion is that it tends to 'predominate' in one's mind; therefore, it will be important to the patient (*Case vignette 2.2*). Cognitive therapy approaches are often indirectly helpful in that the patients get to talk – often for the first time in detail – about their experiences. Open-ended questions such as 'How do you feel?' and 'What are your general problems?' are a good starter, and sympathizing with their beliefs and dilemmas (rather than challenging them, certainly in the first interview or two) can help to elicit more information. This approach does, however, need time, the half an hour or hour of the psychiatric assessment being necessary to get someone to tell you what is on their mind. One very occasionally has to guess, but if patients are not willing to divulge things voluntarily, they will usually say something like 'Not really' or 'I'm not sure'. It is not an easy process for the GP or the specialist (*see also Q 1.16* and *Box 5.1*).

CASE VIGNETTE 2.2

A 59-year-old man was referred by his GP because of constant complaints about his neighbours. His wife had died some 10 years previously and he had been retired for 2 years 'on health grounds'. He was therefore socially isolated, but there was no previous or family history of psychiatric problems. The man was taking a diuretic to treat raised blood pressure but was a non-smoker and non-drinker.

At interview he was pleasant and friendly, neatly dressed and groomed, and quite clear in outlining his concerns. He denied any problems with sleep or appetite, there was no evidence of depressed mood, and there was no evidence that he had any cognitive impairment in terms of limited memory or impaired orientation. He was quite clear, however, that his neighbours were 'interfering with his thoughts'. He believed that they used a word processor to insert thoughts into his mind, and he could also communicate with them via this, assuming that the word processor were switched on. The man insisted that it had to be within a 5-mile radius of his flat in order to work properly.

He also described several auditory hallucinations, of the same people (his neighbours) talking to him in the third person, sometimes saying pleasant things but occasionally being rude. He denied being distressed by them in general but did admit that they had started to interfere with his daily routine of getting up at 8.15 a.m., going shopping, going for a walk and watching television. He was quite convinced that these were real events and was somewhat perplexed as to why his neighbours should be doing this. The man was also willing to take any medication that could help him to sleep and 'relax', and he subsequently responded well to standard antipsychotic agents.

2.23 Are delusions always rather bizarre and strange?

To qualify as the kind of delusion diagnostic of schizophrenia in a formal research sense, delusions have to be bizarre within the patient's social context. It is this very quality which can be so important in defining a belief as a delusion. Such delusions are also not necessarily hard to get out of people, particularly in the early stages of the illness, because they will be a prominent part of the presenting psychopathology. The most commonly missed delusions are, however, those which seem banal, understandable or even semi-real in the patient's social context. A belief that local children do not like you and give you dirty looks probably reflects the reality of a number of individuals anyway. In addition, if they are at all eccentric, they are likely to be picked on – as a local 'nutter' or 'psycho' – so their delusional beliefs will be reinforced by a similar reality. Likewise, the morbidly jealous husband, mistakenly convinced that his partner is having an affair, will not uncommonly drive that partner into an affair by the sheer impossibility of his behaviour. Such delusions, rooted in the day-to-day experience of people's lives, can be difficult to elicit and are more often associated with a delusional disorder (e.g. pure paranoia) than true schizophrenic illness (*see Table 5.5*).

2.24 How do you separate strong religious beliefs or experiences from possible symptoms of schizophrenia?

This is a very delicate question, since the belief that one is the Messiah or Mohammed, for example, or has special religious powers, can be seen as understandable in the light of some religious writings and beliefs. Clarifying patients' roles within their own religious community can be most helpful, by talking to the pastor or priest to see whether there are any oddities that the community itself perceives. Many priests have some experience in terms of understanding mental illness because many mentally ill people come to them for help and they can readily differentiate the intense but genuine believer from the person experiencing psychotic symptoms.

Typical symptoms will include hearing God or the Holy Ghost talking to you, being breathed on or stroked by the Holy Spirit or angels, or believing that you are a special messenger connected up in some special way with the universe, or even the Messiah or Son of God Himself. The main dilemma for such latter figures is their tendency to become public figures of contempt (e.g. David Ikes) or to be publicly mocked or exposed in tabloid headlines. It is noteworthy that such experiences are curiously reminiscent of what seems in fact to have happened to Jesus Christ Himself.

2.25 Do schizophrenic patients have a change in personality or a split personality?

Most families will say that their schizophrenic relative has changed in some way that is quite profound. This will be a blunting of personality, with a lack of drive and interest, or increased eccentricity or oddness. Such changes are typically associated with length of illness and negative symptoms.

The notion of a 'split personality' is entirely incorrect in terms of true schizophrenia. Patients do not suddenly change from being, for example, a gentle giant into a raging beast, unpredictable in terms of what they might do. This sense of distrust is a key feature of the stigma attached to schizophrenia and the butt of many common jokes (e.g. 'You are never alone with schizophrenia').

2.26 Do patients with schizophrenia get disorientated or lose their memory?

Not generally. Schizophrenic symptoms occur in clear consciousness, with no formal impairment of cognition, concentration or memory. Routine mental state examinations should always include a cognitive assessment, and significant cognitive symptoms should make one consider an alternative underlying diagnosis, for example a brain tumour or perhaps alcohol abuse. There is an acknowledged decline in IQ score over time, but this is hard to detect on routine clinical assessment. The one oddity is the tendency of chronic patients to be time-disorientated, old asylum patients regularly insisting that the year they came in is the current year. This may reflect a genuine time disorientation, in that patients feel that they have not grown, changed or had any significant experiences since the year of becoming severely ill. Modern treatments have made this less common as a phenomenon.

2.27 Do patients with schizophrenia always tell you about what is bothering them?

Part of the problem with schizophrenia is eliciting exactly what is going on. The nature of patients' symptoms, the combination of muddled thinking, intermittent hallucinations and a sense of perplexity associated with what is going on can all make it difficult for individuals to give a clear history. They may have complained of being 'depressed' or of not being able to 'concentrate properly'. They sometimes simply stop halfway through a sentence, making the doctor feel frustrated that he or she cannot get to the bottom of things. Complaints may be merely social, related to the neighbours or housing difficulties, or they may be very worried about minor physical symptoms. A particular problem can be trying to distinguish obvious physical illness through this semi-fog of impaired history-giving.

Another difficulty lies in the notion of a 'delusional mood'. This term describes that state of anxiety, like a cloud of uncertainty, which comes on in the early stages of a psychotic breakdown. Patients will feel different or troubled, may experience a sense of being unreal or unnecessarily anxious but will not be able to put their finger on what really is the matter. As the illness progresses, this state of uncertainty seems gradually to coalesce into a distinct delusional belief, and the illness then emerges more clearly. A key feature in managing this kind of illness is to see people regularly in order to gain their trust and clarify their true mental state.

2.28 Is it common in schizophrenia for patients just to seem to smile or laugh to themselves?

Yes. Particularly those patients suffering from hebephrenic schizophrenia seem to have a secret inner world (often called 'autistic') in which they smile, giggle or laugh for no obvious reason. Doctors sometimes feels personally mocked or laughed at because their questions will simply evoke a silly smile or a guffaw of laughter. This symptom is typical of the impaired affect associated with the negative group of symptoms, and some patients even exhibit a so-called 'buffoonery state' in which they seem to act like silly clowns much of the time. It is important to distinguish this from manic depressive illness. If asked why they are laughing, patients often give no reply, but more direct questions, for example 'Do the voices make you laugh?', are often surprisingly successful in establishing symptoms.

2.29 What is meant by anhedonia?

This word derives from the Greek, meaning the opposite of hedonism. That is, it describes a state in which people do not seem to have any particular source of enjoyment or interest. Rather than looking forward to a party, enjoying a film or trying to arrange a holiday, they tend to do very little. This lack of interest in enjoyment needs to be distinguished from the loss of interest and self-blame seen in depressive illness. Anhedonia is one of the most damaging aspects of chronic schizophrenia in that patients find it hard to understand why they should bother to wash, partake in activities or try to make interesting conversation. It is a symptom that probably underlies the sense that many patients, whether in hospital, in day hospital or living independently, seem somehow 'institutionalized' in their behaviour.

2.30 What is meant by the term 'institutionalization'?

Prior to the large-scale closure of the asylums in the 1970s and 80s, there was a genuine concern that patients in hospitals were suffering from 'institutional neurosis', having no choice of what time they got up, what clothes they wore, what they had to eat or what they did during the day. They simply became obedient slaves to the demands of the institution. A number of important studies in the 1950s and 60s seemed to show that there was an enhanced degree of negative symptomatology in patients in asylums where there was little occupational activity, but that more proactive nursing input could genuinely change people's lives and reduce such symptoms.

Although the move to the community has certainly shown that people can live much more independent and personally satisfying lives, there is also evidence that 'institutionalization' reflects in part the chronic negative symptoms (apathy, self-neglect, anhedonia) that are part and parcel of chronic schizophrenia. Getting the right balance between supportive care that is not controlling but not too overstimulating (i.e. if there is excessive emotional expression in the family), so as to drive them into relapse, is an important aspect of ongoing management (*see Box 7.1*).

2.31 Are there really different types of schizophrenia?

As outlined in *Table 2.3*, the current system of classification includes some distinct variants (e.g. paranoid, catatonic) based on different clusters of symptoms. Most clinicians today prefer to consider an individual patient's

---

TABLE 2.3 *ICD-10* classification of types of schizophrenia (section F20)

F20.0	Paranoid	Dominated by (paranoid*) delusions usually with hallucinations (especially auditory); thought disorder obvious in acute states
F20.1	Hebephrenic	Fragmentary delusion/hallucination; mood shallow and inappropriate; mannerisms; disorganized and incoherent speech; solitary; younger patients
F20.2	Catatonic	Prominent psychomotor disturbance, one or more of: stupor/excitement/posturing/negation/waxy flexibility/automatism/perseveration
F20.3	Undifferentiated (atypical)	Active symptoms not conforming to other subtypes
F20.4	Post-schizophrenic depression	Depression +/– some residual schizophrenic symptoms
F20.5	Residual	Chronic negative symptom (deriving from previous psychosis)
F20.6	Simple	Difficult diagnosis; no overt psychosis but declining personal/social function
F20.8 'Other' and F20.9 'Unspecified'		

*Paranoid in this context includes delusions of persecution, reference, exalted birth, special mission, bodily change or jealousy

symptoms as 'positive' or 'negative' (*see Q. 1.20*), using these to monitor treatment or clarify the prognosis. The *ICD-10* categories are mainly useful for research purposes, and many patients will not fit readily into one category. Whether these categories are perhaps different disorders is also uncertain, but every attempt so far to create new diagnoses has failed.

2.32 Are there any worldwide differences in how schizophrenia is formally diagnosed?

The two main systems of classification are currently the 10th edition of the *International Classification of Diseases (ICD-10)* and the 4th edition of the *Diagnostic and Statistical Manual (DSM-IV)*. The former is used largely in Europe, the latter in North America, other countries tending to use one or both, *DSM-IV* probably being more influential. Essentially, as shown in *Table 2.4*, there are not many differences in terms of symptoms, social effects and exclusions. *DSM-IV*, however, requires at least 6 months of illness, compared with the 1 month sufficient for *ICD-10*. By and large therefore, the conditions seen are very similar, but the Americans tend to emphasize chronicity.

TABLE 2.4 Comparison of *ICD-10* and *DSM-IV* diagnostic criteria for schizophrenia

ICD-10	DSM-IV
Symptoms	Symptoms
(At least one clear symptom, or two if less clear cut):	Criterion A
	(Two or more of:)
a) Thought echo/broadcast/withdrawal or insertion	1) Delusions
b) Delusions of control/passivity (including delusional perception)	2) Hallucinations
c) Hallucinations, e.g. running commentary	(only one criterion A symptom is required if delusions are 'bizarre', hallucinations are a running commentary or there are two or more voices)
d) Persistent delusions (culturally inappropriate/impossible)	
(Or at least two symptoms present):	3) Disorganized speech, e.g. incoherence, derailment
a) hallucination in any modality	4) Catatonic/disorganized behaviour
b) broken train of thought → incoherence, neologisms	5) Negative symptoms
c) catatonic behaviours	Criterion B
d) negative symptoms (e.g. apathy, blunting)	For a significant period since the onset of the disturbance, one or more areas of functioning, such as work, interpersonal

TABLE 2.4 Comparison of *ICD-10* and *DSM-IV* diagnostic criteria for schizophrenia—cont'd

ICD-10	DSM-IV
Social factors	relations or self-care are markedly below the level achieved prior to onset
a) Significant and consistent change in the overall quality of some aspects of personal behaviour, manifest as loss of interest, aimlessness, idleness, a self-absorbed attitude and social withdrawal	Criterion C
	Continuous signs of disturbance for at least 6 months; at least 1 month of symptoms meeting Criterion A
Duration	Criterion D
Symptoms clearly present for most of the time during a period of *1 month* or more	1) No major depression; manic or mixed episodes have occurred concurrently with active-phase symptoms
Exclusions	2) If mood episodes occur during active phases, these are only brief relative to the active schizophrenic state
Diagnosis should not be made in the presence of extensive depressive or manic symptoms (unless schizophrenia *antedated* these)	Criterion E
Schizophrenia should not be diagnosed in the presence of overt brain disease or during drug intoxication/withdrawal	Not due to the direct physiological effects of a substance (a drug of abuse, a medication) or a general medical condition

Schizoaffective disorder

If affective *and* schizophrenic symptoms develop together and are evenly balanced ('have occurred concurrently'), a diagnosis of schizoaffective disorder should be made.

PATIENT QUESTIONS

2.33 If someone changes into a different personality, does that mean they have schizophrenia?

Not usually. People who change personality – like Dr Jekyll and Mr Hyde in the famous novel by Robert Louis Stevenson – are rarely schizophrenic. They usually have quite disturbed personality traits, are rather gullible (e.g. they can easily be hypnotized) and have a reason for play-acting different roles, a bit like children who have not grown up. If the changed personality is, however, caused by strange beliefs or experiences such as delusions or hallucinations, with social withdrawal, self-neglect and muddled speech as part of the picture, schizophrenia could well be the reason. Some people even dress up as the opposite sex, complete with wigs and make-up. Again, this is highly unlikely to be due to schizophrenia but relates instead to personality abnormalities, sexual fantasies (transvestism) or even trans-sexualism (the belief you are the wrong gender).

2.34   Is it common to feel that your body has in some way changed?

Yes. Many patients with schizophrenia become quite frightened by lots of different bodily feelings but are often too embarrassed to ask their doctor or tell their families. Sometimes, it seems like a real physical symptom, with pins and needles or even electric shocks in their body or arms, for example. Others feel that their bodies are being distorted or changing shape, or that fluids (or even something alive, like insects or snakes) are moving around inside them. Many people want to have X-rays or brain scans to see what this might be because it feels so real. Others describe their face not looking right or their body feeling like it is made of metal or glass. Some just think that someone is hitting them or biting them, or even stroking them and making them feel aroused. All of these symptoms can be understood as part of the disturbance in the brain and nervous system caused by schizophrenia.

Diagnosis and differential diagnosis

3

3.1 Can you diagnose schizophrenia at a single interview?

If there are direct positive symptoms that can be elicited, and if a patient is cooperative, a reliable diagnosis can be made. The difference between a standard 'new patient' interview by a specialist psychiatrist (between 30 minutes and an hour or more) and with the briefer availabilities of general practice (5–10 minutes) is important here. Diagnosis is also made much easier by the presence of a close relative or friend, enabling one to obtain both a subjective and an objective account of what has been happening. The key features of a *change* and or a *decline* in personal behaviour, the presence of typical symptoms (e.g. hearing voices, experiencing thought block) and the lack of any obvious physical illness are the heart of the matter, the 'royal road' to diagnostic clarity.

3.2 What are the commonest symptoms of schizophrenia?

These are undoubtedly auditory hallucinations (hearing voices) and the various forms of thought disorder. In particular, these include the incoherence associated with thought block, and the sense of perplexity produced by feeling that one's thoughts are controlled, inserted, broadcast, etc. Many patients will also use a phrase like 'I feel depressed' or 'I feel I can't concentrate' in a non-specific way, these feelings being generated by underlying symptoms. A change in behaviour or attitude is also typical, from social confidence to anxious withdrawal, or from reasonable self-care to obvious self-neglect. It is also quite helpful to divide symptoms into 'positive' and 'negative' groups as a means of understanding the illness as well as helping with the appropriate treatment approach (*Table 3.1;* *see also Q. 2.1*).

TABLE 3.1 Positive and negative symptoms of schizophrenia	
Positive	**Negative**
Hallucinations (especially third-person, auditory)	Social withdrawal
Delusions/delusional perception	Flat/incongruous affect
Formal thought disorder	Poverty of speech (alogia)
	Lack of spontaneity (including thought insertion/broadcast/withdrawal)
Passivity experience	Anhedonia/apathy

3.3   Are there typical patterns of symptoms that seem to go together?

Research has shown that are three, relatively common, semi-independent symptom complexes. Although many patients seem to have a condition that is atypical, this being a long-standing problem in terms of relating symptoms to illness course (or even diagnosis) in schizophrenia, the relation between certain symptoms is often worth pursuing. Thus, there seems to be a pattern embraced by the term 'reality distortion', patients being dominated by delusions, hallucinations, passivity and, in essence, a quite florid range of positive symptoms. To the lay person, they are the most obviously unwell in their statements and beliefs.

A second syndrome is termed 'disorganization' because it is characterized by quite active thought disorder with muddled patterns of speech and thinking, and difficulty even saying things. In addition, the relationship between what people say and how they seem to feel (affect) is quite unusual in that they come across as 'silly', blunted or fatuous.

The third group, dominated by negative symptoms and sometimes termed those with 'psychomotor poverty', show social withdrawal, apathy and self-neglect. There is little obviously psychotic about such patients, and they easily get missed because they do not pose any social risk. The term 'Diogenes syndrome' (after Diogenes the Cynic, a 4th century BC philosopher who lived in an earthenware jar and essentially neglected all the usual comforts of life) has been used in some cases to reflect their seeming lack of interest in day-to-day conveniences.

These three syndromes in some way reflect the traditional categories of 'paranoid', 'hebephrenic' and 'simple', but it must again be emphasized that there can be considerable overlap in terms of individual patient presentations (*see Table 2.3*).

3.4   What if the patient has been taking drugs?

There is a strong association between various forms of illicit drug abuse, as well as alcohol dependence, and schizophrenia or similar syndromes.[3] In inner city areas, co-morbidity (i.e. having a schizophrenic illness as well as a degree of drug dependence) has a prevalence of up to 50%. Studies in the USA have shown an increased admission rate with positive cocaine samples in the first few days of the month, that is, in the aftermath of patients receiving their welfare benefits. There is no doubt that schizophrenic symptoms can be exacerbated by drugs and sometimes even mimicked by drug excess in vulnerable individuals.

Common drugs of abuse include cannabis, cocaine (including crack), amphetamines and alcohol. There is a debate about the role of cannabis in that it seems to exacerbate some patients' presentations, while making others feel simply 'mellow' and in fact helping them get through the day. Cocaine and especially amphetamines are, in terms of their dopamine-stimulant activity, clearly likely to bring on a relapse and can quickly exacerbate symptoms. Routine drug screening, via urine or even hair samples, may be necessary to clarify what is going on (*Table 3.2*).

TABLE 3.2 Drugs typically associated with schizophrenia-like symptoms

Drug	Symptoms
Cannabis (tetrahydrocannabinol)	May enhance paranoid/hallucinatory experiences (or may calm/lower arousal)
Amphetamines*	Paranoid delusions, auditory (and other) hallucinations, agitation, hostility
Cocaine (and crack cocaine)*	Agitation, tactile/auditory hallucinations, paranoid thinking
LSD/ecstasy/mescaline (peyote)/ magic mushrooms (psilocybin)**	Confusional/hallucinatory (visual) state of brief (1–3 days') duration, euphoria, insomnia
Alcohol	Withdrawal state includes visual hallucinations, delirium and paranoid ideation
Benzodiazepines	Withdrawal state includes hallucination, agitation and sense of bodily distortion
Dopamine agonists (e.g. anti-parkinsonian medication)*	
Steroids	Variable effects, including psychotic or manic symptoms, confusion and agitation
Ketamine/phenylcyclidine (PCP)***	Distorted body image, excitation, hallucinations (various) and delusions

*Act via dopamine receptor; **act via serotonin receptor; ***act via glutamate receptor

3.5   What do we mean by 'first-rank symptoms'?

As outlined in *Table 2.1*, this was a term used by the leading German psychopathologist Kurt Schneider to define those kinds of symptom that he considered were diagnostic of schizophrenia. If one of these was elicited, he considered that the patient really had a schizophrenic illness. However, he also considered that symptoms of the 'second rank', if there were enough, could make up for the absence of first-rank symptoms, and still clinch the diagnosis. This is partly acknowledged in the *ICD-10*[4] and *DSM-IV* classifications, particularly when negative symptoms, social decline and a change in personality are the main presenting features.

3.6 If a patient has just one symptom, is that enough to call it schizophrenia?

There has long been a debate about how many symptoms are needed to clinch the diagnosis, but is generally accepted that a true first-rank symptom, if held for more than a few days (at least a month in most categorizations), is indicative of schizophrenic illness. A number of patients seem, however, to have just one symptom, for example hearing voices, and literally nothing else. They do not decline personally, they maintain social relationships, they dress and act normally, and in various ways they cope with their symptoms. Thus, in a long-term study following up a cohort of patients, over 10% were stable and on no medication even though they had been really quite ill when first diagnosed. It should also be understood that just having one delusional belief is part and parcel of what is now called 'delusional disorder' but used to be called 'paranoia' (see below).

3.7 Should families be in on the initial interview with a patient?

It is an accepted truth that a corroborative history, from someone who knows the patient well, is vital in clarifying the diagnosis. Patients who are severely unwell cannot, by definition, give a clear history; their recall of events may be dominated by the nature of their symptoms, or they may be embarrassed and wish to cover up what has really been happening. If patients refuse to have anyone else around (confidentiality being a core issue here), the doctor has a dilemma. Asking the patient whether the family can be involved is very much part of good management. If there are genuine risks, to the patient's health or to public safety, because of the nature of a patient's symptoms, confidentiality can clearly be outweighed by the need to reduce risk. Contacting the family in this context is of course a priority.

If the initial assessment of the patient can be made with a member of the family (or close friend) present, much more can be obtained, and a quicker diagnosis and treatment programme can be undertaken. Confidentiality issues can easily be used to avoid taking difficult decisions in treatment, and getting the balance right between care and neglect is not always easy.

3.8 What if families and patients disagree over what's been going on?

This is not uncommon in that paranoid patients will insist that their mother, for example, is just 'exaggerating' or has got 'the wrong end of the stick'. The situation is most complex if one is concerned that both the patient *and* the family member might be unwell! The principles of management involve assessing the patient's mental state and history, to whatever degree one can, and trying to get an independent assessment from the family. Involving a third party, a friend or a neighbour, may be vital to the process of pinning down just what is going on. In this context, a GP or other professional who knows the patient and family well can be a vital link in clarifying the differences.

Essentially, if the pattern of symptoms elicited by one party is typical of the diagnosis, it is most likely that schizophrenia is occurring. The scenario of people making up symptoms, as if out of a cookbook, for malicious purposes is largely confined to the movies.

3.9 Can one diagnose schizophrenia if the patient has no obvious 'first-rank' symptoms?

Yes. Even though there is no evidence that they are obviously psychotic (i.e. expressing delusions or experiencing hallucinations), a number of patients have so clearly changed that schizophrenia must be high on the list of differential diagnoses. This may be a behavioural change, in terms of social withdrawal, lack of self-care or an impaired level of communication. Difficulty understanding or clarifying patients' statements or concerns, an obvious difference reported in their social behaviour and the clear indication, from those who know them, that they have 'changed' or are 'not themselves' are highly typical. When one explores the background more closely, evidence will often emerge that some genuine first-rank symptoms were experienced but had for some reason been overlooked.

3.10 Can the GP do any blood tests that can help with a differential diagnosis?

These are outlined in *Table 3.3* – a number of very important, basic investigations can help to exclude alternative causes for a schizophrenia-like presentation. Since common diseases occur commonly, there is a high likelihood that these tests will prove unhelpful, and diagnosis must therefore be based on the mental state examination and history, the essence of good psychiatric practice. Nevertheless, a full blood count with erythrocyte sedimentation rate to exclude infections or unusual metabolic conditions such as systemic lupus erythematosus, liver function tests to help exclude underlying alcoholism, and thyroid function tests, particularly in older people, are worth doing routinely. Anything else should be based on the symptoms or signs found on examination. A urinary drug screen, which is now readily available and quite comprehensive for the whole range of recreational/illicit drugs, should also be routine.

TABLE 3.3 Differential diagnosis of schizophrenia

Test	Possible differential diagnosis
Full blood count	Anaemia (?HIV); raised mean corpuscular volume indicating vitamin B12 deficiency or alcohol abuse; underlying infection (raised white cell count)
Erythrocyte sedimentation rate	Chronic illness (e.g. tuberculosis); autoimmune disorder (e.g. systemic lupus erythematosus)
Liver function tests	Evidence of alcohol-induced abnormality (e.g. raised gamma-glutamyl transaminase) or uncommon metabolic disorder (e.g. Wilson's disease – excessive copper deposition)
Thyroid function tests	Evidence of hypo- or hyper-thyroidism; the former can present with paranoid psychotic symptoms, the latter with anxiety/agitation
?Early morning blood cortisol level	If signs of endocrine abnormality

3.11 What physical illnesses can present with schizophrenia-like symptoms?

If one excludes the effects of drugs, either recreational or prescribed (e.g. steroids), physical illnesses can generally be categorized into unusual infections, forms of brain or neurological damage and metabolic conditions. The classic differential diagnosis is temporal lobe epilepsy, the symptoms of which typically include visual, auditory and olfactory hallucinations, an episodic course and quite unusual behaviour. Any head injuries and a number of rarer hereditary conditions (e.g. Huntington's chorea or porphyria, especially of acute type), also need sometimes to be excluded. It should be emphasized that these are generally the exception and can readily be eliminated from the differential diagnosis by good history-taking (*Table 3.4*).

3.12 How can one differentiate between schizophrenia and depression?

This is often difficult, patients commonly saying that they feel 'depressed' or describing other depressive symptoms, for example poor sleep, suicidal ideation and loss of concentration. It is thus vital to ask what individual patients mean by the term 'depression', getting them to explain their state of mind. Useful questions in this regard might be 'How does depression affect you?' and 'What makes you think you are depressed?' Truly depressed patients will be slowed down, will blame themselves and will generally be older. Schizophrenic patients will be (at least at first onset) in their late teens or early 20s, will tend to find external reasons for their experiences and will show a degree of perplexity that is not typical of true depression. The oldest rule in the book, however, is that if one is uncertain of the diagnosis, patients under 40 are more likely to have schizophrenia, or something within that range of illnesses, whereas those over 40 are more likely to have depression.

TABLE 3.4 Physical illnesses associated with schizophrenia-like presentations or symptoms*

Group	Disorder	Symptoms
Epilepsy	Especially temporal lobe	Olfactory/visual hallucinations
Infectious conditions	HIV, encephalitis/meningo-encephalitis, neurosyphilis ('general paralysis of the insane'), cysticercosis, other tropical diseases/infestations, e.g. cerebral malaria and typhoid fever	Non-specific, half-formed delusions and/or hallucinations
Brain injury	Acute or chronic, trauma (acute or chronic)	Non-specific half-formed delusions and / or hallucinations
Stroke (cerebro-vascular accident)	Or cerebrovascular abnormalities as well as accidents	Sometimes location specific, e.g. visual hallucinations if is occipital lobe damage
Neurological disorders	Multiple sclerosis, Schilder's disease, metachromatic leukodystrophy	Non-specific
Rare conditions	Huntington's chorea, Wilson's disease, porphyria (especially acute), homocystinuria	Non-specific
Metabolic/endocrine	Systemic lupus erythematosus, hypothyroidism, excessive steroids (natural or prescribed)	Paranoid delusions

*Most of these conditions can also be a cause of manic symptoms

3.13 Do patients with schizophrenia show abnormalities on IQ testing?

Not usually. There is no evidence that patients with schizophrenia, at least in terms of a first onset, have any formal cognitive impairments such as would be picked up by a standard IQ test, for example the Wechsler Adult Intelligence Scale. However, the prevalence of schizophrenia seems to be some 2–3 times greater in people with learning difficulties (which fits with the general theory of some form of diffuse brain damage), and formal testing may be useful to clarify the background IQ. There is, not uncommonly, a degree of decline in IQ over 5–10 years. Neither the overall result nor the resulting subtest scores will have any diagnostic relevance, but they can be useful in clarifying the extent to which a significant learning difficulty also handicaps an individual patient. In terms of the provision of services, they can also be useful to clarify whether the learning difficulty or the schizophrenia (or schizophrenia-like symptoms) is the key problem so that the appropriate specialist team for continuing care can be assigned.

3.14 Are any particular psychological tests or scales useful in diagnosis?

There are no formal psychological tests (outside the research environment) that can provide the core diagnosis of schizophrenia. This remains based on obtaining the appropriate history, on a good mental state examination and (if necessary) on observation and continued review over a period of time as an inpatient and/or outpatient. There are, however, a number of rating scales that can usefully establish the severity of the illness and help in evaluating, at least in a formal sense, when people are getting better, for example during drug trials.

These scales include the Brief Psychiatric Rating Scale (*Appendix 1*), which simply looks at symptoms (and their severity on a scale of 1 to 4), and standard research assessments such as the SAPS and SANS (scales for the assessment of positive/negative symptoms), the Present State Examination and the Positive and Negative Symptoms Scale. Scales have also been developed for social functioning and quality of life, and the use of questionnaires in general in the management of schizophrenia is increasingly recognized as making assessment and treatment plans more reliable (see also *References* and *Further reading*).

3.15 Should one always do an EEG (electroencephalogram)?

It is generally accepted that an EEG is not a necessary, routine investigation. Unless there is obvious evidence, from the history or examination, of an ictal disorder (i.e. episodic changes in behaviours that seem like fits, or evidence of blackouts), the likelihood of any abnormality emerging on the EEG is extremely low. Furthermore, even if EEG findings are negative, one still cannot exclude an epileptic condition (*Case vignette 3.1*). Only if there is a clear observation of unusual behaviours of an intermittent type, for example sudden falls or what look like fits, should one consider an EEG. Nevertheless, pressure from patients and families may require that such investigations (as well as other tests such as computed tomography (CT) brain scans) are carried out in order to make them feel that everything has been done to exclude a physical condition.

CASE VIGNETTE 3.1

A 27-year-old woman was referred by her GP because of 'strange attacks' in the context of what seemed to be a typical schizophrenic illness. This had been characterized by auditory hallucinations (voices that commented on her actions) and by beliefs that people were following her, coming into her house and stealing things, and at times spraying her with an unpleasant smell. She had taken appropriate medication but continued to have 'strange attacks'.

On further review, she described at times a sense of a bad smell making her eyes lose focus. She then would experience objects becoming bright and sharp, and changing colour and size. The woman also experienced déjà vu phenomena, a sense of perplexity and a sense of being looked at and even threatened by the way people looked at her. Such episodes tended to last anything up to an hour or more, and she insisted that she was 'completely fine' between them.

In view of these symptoms, and with no other abnormalities in terms of mental state examination, physical assessment or special investigations, including a CT scan and EEG, consideration was given to her experiencing a form of temporal lobe epilepsy. It was agreed that she should start on a combination of carbamazepine and an antipsychotic agent, which led to a significant improvement in this lady's mental state over the course of the next 6 months. Despite repeated EEGs, no evidence of a formal epileptic abnormality was found, and she continued to experience occasional episodes of 'bad smells', which rarely progressed to anything more distressing.

3.16 Is it worth doing a CT or magnetic resonance imaging brain scan in a young person in particular?

Given an appropriate history and mental state examination, the diagnosis is unlikely to be clarified by the use of either of these investigations, although they are helpful as part of research studies, and there is evidence that patients with schizophrenia tend to have a greater likelihood of certain abnormalities, for example enlarged ventricles. These changes are, however, non-specific, and significant differences emerge only with reasonably large research cohorts. Such findings do indicate therefore that there is an underlying brain disorder, with loss of brain tissue to some degree in many patients, but routinely carrying out such a scan is not justified. Again, if the patient or family is very worried about a brain disorder or brain tumour, it is only humane to try to demonstrate to them that there is no abnormality. This may be an important aspect of dealing with the stigma and non-compliance associated with the refusal to accept that one has a 'psychiatric' diagnosis.

If there is an obvious neurological abnormality, or an obvious history of head injury or other cerebral insult, a scan is mandatory.

3.17 How can you differentiate drug abuse from schizophrenia?

The use of routine urine drug screens, in all new or relapsed patients, is now standard practice in most psychiatric units. These are highly sensitive and pick up all the usual recreational drugs. The drugs most commonly associated with pseudo-schizophrenia-like syndromes are amphetamine sulphate ('speed') and, to a lesser extent, ecstasy (MDMA), lysergic acid diethylamide (LSD) and cocaine. It is also worth remembering that a number of prescribed drugs (e.g. steroids, and dopamine agonists for Parkinsonism) can in themselves cause psychotic symptoms. Thus, apart from a urine drug screen (if patients let you), getting hold of all the medications they have been prescribed and obtaining a corroborative history (from friends perhaps more than parents) can help. It should also be remembered that because a person tests positive, especially for cannabis (widely used now among young people, especially in inner cities), it does not mean that is the cause of their condition. The evidence for genuine cannabis-induced schizophrenia remains very thin, although high doses of tetrahydrocannabinol (THC), the active ingredient of cannabis, can lead to toxic effects that have a psychotic quality (*see also Table 3.2, Table 4.2, and Q. 4.7, 4.8, 5.2 and 5.26*).

3.18 What is the best way of screening for illicit drugs?

This can be done by urine testing, hair testing or direct questioning. The former is most widely used, relatively simple and reasonably sensitive. Shorter-acting drugs (e.g. cocaine) will, however, disappear from the urine within approximately 24–48 hours, whereas cannabis remains for a number of days. Taking the urine sample as near as possible to the acute presentation is most important.

Hair samples are much more sensitive over a longer period of time, drugs accumulating in the hair as it grows. They are now increasingly being used for routine monitoring, for example of drug-dependent patients or patients in specific legal programmes. Dipstick preparations are also now available for direct in-surgery use on urine samples or for relatives and friends to use at home.

3.19 Are families good at recognizing illness in their relatives?

Most families know quite quickly that something has happened. They will describe a change in behaviour, a change in personality, social withdrawal ('He keeps staying in his room, doctor') and a sense of concern over odd remarks or a changed pattern of dress. There is clearly a problem with adolescent patients, given the usual variegations of teenage styles of dressing, behaving and speaking. Families with a history of schizophrenia in their background (e.g. a mother who 'had a breakdown' or a grandfather who was 'in a mental hospital') may be much more sensitized to the dilemmas and much more ready to see illness symptoms in adolescents or young adults who do not quite seem to conform to expectations.

On the other hand, the stigma of the illness leads to many families denying what is quite obvious. They may believe that it must be because of drugs or because someone has spiked their son's drink, or they may blame his school for poor management. Some will insist on only using terms such as 'depressed' and 'troubled', and ask for counselling rather than treatment. Assessing the family's awareness of and insight into the nature of the illness is a key part of the management of schizophrenia. Some behaviour patterns typical of – but *not* diagnostic of – schizophrenic illnesses are outlined in *Table 3.5*.

3.20 Should you always get a specialist opinion when you think there is a diagnosis of schizophrenia?

In general, yes, for two reasons. First, the average GP will only see about 10–15 new schizophrenic patients in the course of a lifetime's practice, in contrast to the average consultant psychiatrist, who probably sees one or two a month. Although obvious illnesses are not difficult to diagnose, masked ones (that look like depression or adolescent angst) are. Second, the social and treatment complexities of an illness such as schizophrenia, with its likely long-term consequences and the associated stigma, usually mean that specialist care is likely to be needed. Non-acceptance or denial of the diagnosis, by patient or family, will also require consultant help, sooner rather than later. Specialist investigations, or even hospital admission in order to clarify matters, are often necessary at the beginning of an illness.

3.21 Can any prescribed medications cause or exacerbate schizophrenic symptoms?

Psychological reactions to drug treatment are not uncommon but are difficult to quantify. Feeling tired or slowed down can mimic depression, whereas medications that cause arousal reactions (e.g. increased pulse rate, sweating and difficulty sleeping) can lead to anxiety or panic attacks. Old people in particular are prone to confusional states, particularly if given too

TABLE 3.5 Unusual behaviours distinctive in (but not diagnostic of) schizophrenia*

Behaviour	Meaning
Ear plugs, head coverings and hoods	Trying to exclude intrusive hallucinations or sense of thought insertion or interference from passers-by
Windows covered up (e.g. with blankets)	To exclude intrusive hallucinations or due to a sense of being spied on or interfered with
Staying indoors (especially by day)	Withdrawing from other people who may represent a threat, a source of 'voices', a source of physical discomfort or a deliberate distortion of one's lifestyle
Unusual postures/gestures	A response to command hallucinations, or being generated by somatic delusions, e.g. keeping still in order to avoid your body breaking up, as if it were made of glass
Broken/rejected television	The television is peculiarly intrusive because of its combination of audio and visual inputs – people on television are seen as giving personal messages or as a source of voices, inserted thoughts, etc.
Excessive washing/cleaning	To get rid of supposed dirt, miasma, smell or 'noxious gas' imposed on one's environment. May include obsession-like rituals to wash away germs, body odour or unseen fleas/lice

*These may well, for several months or more, precede overt symptoms during onset or relapse. Relatives quickly come to recognize them after quite subtle behavioural changes and should be supported in their concerns.

high a dosage, and fleeting hallucinations or paranoid ideas can be associated with such reactions. Disorders with a fleeting or intermittent resemblance to schizophrenia, for example because someone is hallucinating, can often fluctuate with mood changes or disorientation. The two types of medication most closely associated with psychotic symptoms are dopamine agonists and steroids (*see Table 3.2*), this effect often being dose related.

Rarer reactions that are worth bearing in mind are listed in *Table 3.6*. The two best documented groups of drug are appetite suppressants, particularly dexamphetamine (although others of its class can have such a reaction) and antimalarial drugs such as mefloquine (Lariam). Checking closely the names and doses of the patient's medications, particularly when people are taking a large combination of medications, is good practice in this regard.

3.22 Does schizophrenia come on in any particular age group?

It is generally accepted that schizophrenia is an illness of young people, onset between the ages of 18 and 28 being most likely. It is also true that the illness tends to come on at a younger age in men than in women, although

TABLE 3.6 Medications associated with psychotic symptoms (e.g. hallucinations) as a side-effect (usually rare but worth bearing in mind)

Group	Drug	Comment
Gastrointestinal	H$_2$-Receptor antagonists, e.g. cimetidine; appetite suppressants, e.g. phentermine; dexamfetamine (significant problem)	Especially problematic in the elderly or very ill
Cardiorespiratory	Ephedrine; digoxin; procainamide	Dose related
Anticonvulsants	Vigabatrin; topiramate; ethosuximide	Also depression, mania, agitation and concentration problems. Also depression and euphoria
Analgesics	Tramadol; nabilone; opioids; nefopam	Hallucinations and confusion; mood changes
Treatment of alcohol dependence	Disulfiram (Antabuse)	All forms of psychosis
Treatment of infections	Cycloserine (anti-tuberculous) Dapsone (anti-leprotic) Quinolones, e.g. ofloxacin (for urinary tract infections), mefloquine (Lariam), chloroquine	Discontinue as soon as possible (significant problem)
	Antiviral agents, e.g. ganciclovir, Foscarnet sodium, famciclovir, aciclovir	Hallucinations, confusion and agitation

N.B. This is not an exhaustive list but is derived from the side-effects listed in the British National Formulary the reasons for this are not clear. Thus, the average age of onset in males is about 22 or 23 years, but in females about 26 or 27 years. Onset in teenagers (14–16 years) is also well known and unfortunately tends to have a poorer prognosis because of the impairments in personality development. A later onset, in one's 40s or 50s, tends to be more common in women than men but is often preceded by a history of idiosyncratic, eccentric or socially isolative behaviours (*see Fig. 3.1*).

3.23 Is schizophrenia commoner in any particular cultural or racial group?

One of the unique aspects of schizophrenia is that its prevalence seems roughly the same wherever one is in the world (roughly, between 0.5% and 0.8%). Two large World Health Organization field surveys[1,5] using standardized rating scales and clear diagnostic criteria have shown that symptoms, incidence and prevalence do not vary much, whether in

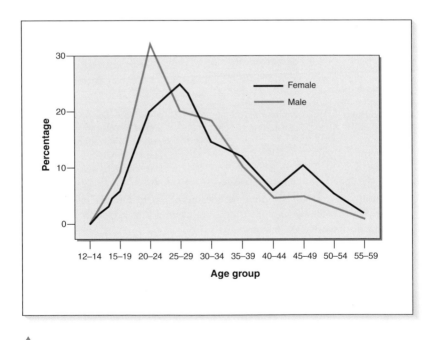

Fig. 3.1 Age and sex distribution of schizophrenia (defined as age of onset of psychotic symptoms or first hospitalization). Note the bimodal age at onset pattern for females. From Cannon, M 2002 Schizophrenia: Epidemiology and Risk Factors *Psychiatry*: 2002 1: 9. By kind permission of The Medicine Publishing Company

developed or developing countries, north or south, hot or cold. There are some apparent exceptions to this, which can probably be explained by emigration or selective breeding, and *Figure 3.2* illustrates how definitions can narrow the incidence range reported.

Among native Taiwanese (i.e. not the large numbers who fled mainland China to Taiwan during the Communist takeover) and in the Hutterite religious sect in South Dakota, for example, the rate seems to be lower. By contrast, small areas in the West of Ireland and Northern Sweden seem to have higher rates, whereas especially higher rates (four to sixfold increases) have been reported among second-generation African-Caribbean immigrants into the UK. Particular concern, related to fears of racism and misdiagnosis, has been expressed about this group. However, most immigrant groups have an increased rate of mental illness, for reasons that are not always clear. In the case of the African-Caribbeans, problems with the census (i.e. people not registering), selective migration and the cultural misinterpretation of manic or depressive symptoms may provide some of the answers. It is notable that third-generation African-Caribbeans do not seem to show an increased incidence, whereas the rate amongst South Asian immigrants actually seems lower.

Given the essentially similar prevalence of schizophrenia in the countries of origin of all these immigrant groups, it is, however, highly likely that the reported differences are essentially social artefacts. The ability of families, for example, to cover up embarrassing conditions, or the absence of a family, may make all the difference. Likewise, cultural responses to symptoms, whether shy withdrawal or externalized agitation, can lower or enhance the recognizability of a disorder.

3.24 Is misdiagnosis common when it comes to schizophrenia?

Not usually. Reliability ratings are, for appropriately trained clinicians, of the order of 0.8 (i.e. about 80% or more). This is better than, for example, the reliability of diagnosis of an acute abdomen, and in this sense psychiatric assessment, despite relying on mental state examination and history-taking (rather than blood tests and X-rays), is, in terms of psychoses such as schizophrenia, usually quite accurate. Studies reviewing changing diagnoses in different individuals tend to show a move towards, rather than away from, schizophrenia. It is thus not uncommon for an initial diagnosis, especially in a young person, of 'personality disorder', 'drug-induced psychosis' or even 'depression', to be changed to schizophrenia over the course of the next 2 or 3 years (*Case vignette 3.2*). The reverse is, however, rarely true, although drug-induced states, the extreme paranoia of some people's agoraphobia and forms of personality disorder (especially if coloured by drugs and/or alcohol) can make diagnosis difficult. Because of the stigma, long-term consequences and treatment needs for patients with

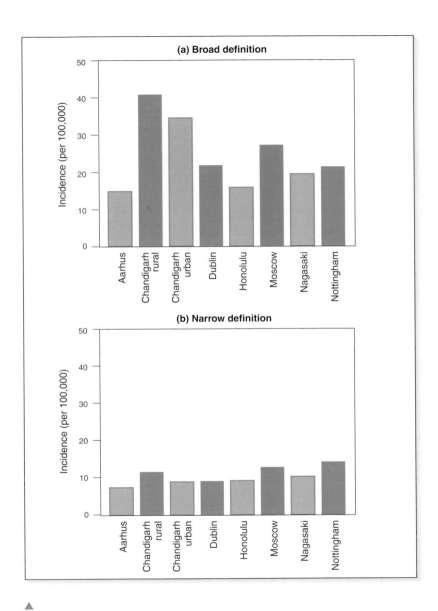

▲

Fig. 3.2 Geographical variations in the incidence of schizophrenia (a) broadly defined and (b) narrowly defined. Data from the International Pilot Study of Schizophrenia[1]. Note that, subsequent studies have demonstrated differing results, suggesting higher rates in certain immigrant groups and among those born or brought up in urban areas (*see Fig. 4.5*).

schizophrenia, most psychiatric teams are very careful in evaluating patients fully before coming to a conclusive diagnosis.

CASE VIGNETTE 3.2

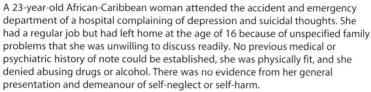

A 23-year-old African-Caribbean woman attended the accident and emergency department of a hospital complaining of depression and suicidal thoughts. She had a regular job but had left home at the age of 16 because of unspecified family problems that she was unwilling to discuss readily. No previous medical or psychiatric history of note could be established, she was physically fit, and she denied abusing drugs or alcohol. There was no evidence from her general presentation and demeanour of self-neglect or self-harm.

On being reviewed by the psychiatric team, who arranged outpatient as well as home treatment assessments and support, this lady gradually divulged more of her concerns. She talked of her sense of isolation over the previous 2–3 years and her sense that she could not get on in her work because of 'racist attitudes'. She admitted to poor sleep, some difficulty in concentrating and difficulty making friends. Her manner was generally tearful and depressed, and she denied any unusual experiences, such as hearing voices. She was started on an antidepressant and offered crisis admission – into a supportive crisis house for women of her background rather than a hospital ward – if it were required.

The patient initially seemed to respond to treatment, becoming less anxious, denying suicidal thoughts and even returning part time to work. It was nevertheless difficult to obtain background information, and she had only recently registered with her GP so there was also no readily available primary care history. Her family were in fact in another part of the country, and she was unwilling to have them contacted. Because of her gradual improvement, and her concerns about having a 'psychiatric' label, the crisis team withdrew, and continuing care was provided by her GP.

Some 2 months later, she presented once more in a somewhat confused state. She now felt that the racist attitudes at work had become worse and even described people making unpleasant comments about her, for example that she smelt. The patient was unwilling to come to hospital but was prepared to go to the crisis unit, where she was closely monitored. She became more guarded and, although denying suicidal ideation, was noted to be isolating herself more and more. An urgent psychiatric assessment was requested. At a home visit, her obvious agitation, the fact that she was now clearly responding to hallucinations (auditory) and the delusional nature of her beliefs about other people (not only were they 'racist', but they were also deliberately following her and 'making faces' at her in public) indicated that she had developed clear schizophrenic symptoms. She was admitted under Section 2 of the Mental Health Act because of the risks to her own health, as evidenced by her suicidal intent.

In hospital, she responded well to an atypical antipsychotic agent, along with supportive counselling and a psychoeducation programme aimed at improving insight. The patient was, however, still unwilling for her family to be contacted, and maintaining support after discharge was impeded by her wishing to move away. She did not give her move-on address, but 3 months later contact was made by another community mental health team, who were confidentially advised of her relevant history and symptoms. She had made a serious suicidal attempt, by hanging, and had been readmitted to hospital. The lady's cultural beliefs and family attitudes had made it very difficult for her to accept she had schizophrenia, and she felt herself to be demeaned by the 'label'.

3.25 Are other mental illnesses commonly misdiagnosed as schizophrenia?

In general the diagnosis of schizophrenia, based on reliable criteria, is in itself reliable. However, a number of other conditions do have overlapping symptoms, and clinicians generally try to delay confirming a schizophrenic diagnosis, because of its implications and (especially in the early stages of the disorder) the similarity to forms of depression or drug-induced states. Many patients will have been described as depressed or anxious prior to their schizophrenic illness becoming quite obvious, while difficult patients may be labelled as suffering from a 'personality disorder' because of the behavioural problems in management. Key areas of the differential diagnosis between schizophrenia and other psychiatric disorders are outlined in *Table 3.7*.

3.26 How can you confirm the diagnosis of schizophrenia?

There is no definitive blood test, radiological investigation or physical sign that is absolutely – 100% – diagnostic of schizophrenia. However, the presence of established symptoms, especially 'first-rank' symptoms (*see Table 2.1*), the absence of any other cause for changes in behaviour or social decline, and the typical history of a given patient are all powerful clues, with considerable reliability. In more difficult states, it may take several years, or even longer, to decide on the diagnosis as symptoms evolve. A trial of treatment may also be quite informative in that the obvious response to antipsychotics, in terms of behaviour, communication, self-care and improved social stability, is in itself indicative of an underlying psychotic process.

3.27 How often do patients pretend to have schizophrenic symptoms (pseudo-psychosis)?

A common problem, for accident and emergency departments in particular, is the presentation of someone complaining of voices who seems to be trying to manipulate an admission. In the era of risk management, this makes for considerable difficulties, most duty psychiatrists preferring to admit and review rather than argue with difficult patients or demanding friends and relatives. Such patients will usually be those with true schizophrenia, emphasizing the voices because of their own state of distress, isolation or impoverishment (benefits having run out), or patients with forms of personality disorder (often associated with alcohol or drug abuse), whose 'voices' are essentially internal voice-like thoughts that make them feel bad. Unless patients are well known, a differential diagnosis in the acute situation is very difficult. Every GP and psychiatric department has its collection of highly dependent patients, who exaggerate or add to their symptoms, or even mimic other patients' symptoms. Experienced nurses will recognize this, and it is interesting how certain phrases or experiences suddenly emerge in patients of uncertain diagnosis after they have been in contact with established schizophrenics (*see also Q. 5.20* and *5.21*).

The deliberate feigning of symptoms, as in Munchausen's syndrome, overlaps this but is very rare in those who do not have some other form of mental illness anyway. Formal pseudo-psychosis, however, describes those patients who present with true symptoms and then subsequently state that they were only putting them on. This may be days or weeks later, often after treatment. Such patients unfortunately tend to have a bad prognosis, the claims of pretence being indicative of very poor insight and probable non-compliance with future treatment.

3.28 Can one really diagnose schizophrenia, or is it just a label for people who are a bit different?

The reliability of a schizophrenic diagnosis has been well established, across cultures and countries, by a number of studies. Thus, given a particular pattern of symptoms, course and exclusions, a quite coherent picture emerges. The pattern of symptoms can also point to who will respond to treatment, which is the point of the diagnostic exercise in the first place. The lack of blood tests, radiological investigations or even biopsies that can provide organic confirmation does not mean that the diagnosis is invalid but only that future research will tell.

It is also worth considering how one would expect a disorder of brain function (as opposed to structure) to present. Given that the brain is the organ that provides thoughts, ideas and emotions, that handles one's perceptual apparatus (e.g. hearing and seeing) and that connects all of this with bodily function, the pattern of symptoms of schizophrenia could be expected if there were brain dysfunction. Thus, getting the wrong idea (delusion) or hearing something that is not there (hallucination) can be seen as the logical abnormalities to be expected from a malfunctioning brain.

3.29 What is the difference between schizophrenia and a delusional disorder?

Whereas schizophrenia is an illness with a number of symptoms, usually coming on in young people and involving obvious decline or a change in how someone presents, delusional disorder (formerly known as pure 'paranoia') is much less obvious. Apart from patients having one single delusion – which might be a delusional system, for example that Freemasons are constantly interfering with their life and delaying promotion at work (with many complex instances of how this is done) –

there is no other obvious impairment. Patients are appropriately dressed and groomed, live overtly normal lives, are quite coherent and almost never experience any kind of hallucination. Onset is usually in middle age, the delusion often being related to someone's life situation, for example persecutory delusions in members of minority groups, and there are usually no mood symptoms, although depression can sometimes intervene because of difficulties that the patient faces. The whole process comes on gradually, often over months or years, the delusion increasingly dominating the person's life.

The content varies, but there is often a constant sense of being persecuted (in business or at home). It can just be a system of morbid jealousy (e.g. about a spouse) or can involve litigation. There is in fact a legal classification – the querulous litigant – which enables judges to ban people from taking on any more legal actions, on the grounds that they are wasting the court's time. It may be a physical belief, about your body being misshapen or believing that people think you smell. Most patients have very poor insight, the condition tends to drag on and on, and they often end up as isolated and embittered eccentrics, whose friends and family have backed away in exasperation (*Table 3.7*).

3.30 What is the difference between schizophrenia and schizotypal disorder?

The category of schizotypal disorder (in *ICD-10*) is somewhat controversial and has in the past been called 'borderline' or 'latent' schizophrenia. Another term used was 'pseudo-neurotic' schizophrenia, and there seems to be a considerable overlap with schizoid or paranoid personality disorders. It is a kind of half-way house between a full-blown schizophrenia and a self-isolating style of personality, and patients often have a family member with full schizophrenia. It is thus considered to be part of the genetic 'spectrum' of schizophrenia.

Symptoms include a rather aloof manner, poor social skills with others, somewhat odd beliefs, with a degree of suspiciousness, a tendency to ruminate and be somewhat vague and circumstantial, and (occasionally) transient, near-psychotic episodes, for example illusions or delusion-like ideas. The condition tends to rumble on, a more full-blown schizophrenic illness sometimes emerging after several years (*see Table 3.7*).

3.31 Is there any particular pattern of childhood behaviour that can help in the diagnosis?

Research has increasingly shown that certain childhood styles, or patterns of behaviour, are seen in patients (especially boys) who subsequently develop schizophrenia. Unfortunately, these remain largely non-specific, so while most schizophrenic patients will have caused concern (to the family or school) in their childhood years, possibly even attending a child guidance unit, there will be a lot of 'noise' in the system. Reviews of home videos in America are fascinating in showing how the pre-schizophrenic child seems to stand apart from the social group at parties, for example, and mothers often report that they were 'different' from other children. Impaired social contact, difficulties relating to other children at school, impaired motor or speech development and enhanced anxiety are also commonly reported. All these behaviours can, however, be associated with other factors as well so although providing hints, they are not diagnostic or definitely predictive. If there is a pattern of social avoidance, unusual behaviours in public and a strong family history of inherited schizophrenia (*see also Q. 4.2, 4.19* and *9.2*), close monitoring of such a child is clearly justified. Possible childhood precursors are summarized in *Table 3.8*.

TABLE 3.7 Differential diagnoses of schizophrenia and other psychiatric disorders

Disorder	Similarities	Differences
Mania	Agitation, incoherence, hallucinations, delusions	Flight of ideas vs thought disorders Mood-congruent delusions (usually grandiose) On/off course
Depression	Withdrawn, 'negative symptoms', retardation	Older age group, no 'first-rank' symptoms, self blame
Drug-induced psychoses, alcohol dependence/ withdrawal	Paranoid delusions, hallucinations, agitated	Brief onset and course (hours to days) Visual distortions +/- 'confusion' Tremor, sweats, delirium
Personality disorders	Unusual behaviours, paranoid ideation, apparent 'voices'	No 'first-rank' symptoms Inconsistent presentations Often drug or alcohol related
Panic syndrome/ agoraphobia	Ideas of reference, (?delusional) agitation, paranoid thinking	No 'first-rank' symptoms Other typical panic/ anxiety symptoms
Delusional disorder	Delusions or delusional system	Later onset No other psychotic symptoms 'Normal' social presentation
Schizotypal disorder	Eccentric/withdrawn, transient perceptual abnormalities	No persisting psychotic symptoms No clear onset or decline

TABLE 3.8 Possible childhood precursors of schizophrenia

Social	Anxiety/increased sensitivity in social situations (self-report)
	Preferring to play alone
	Fewer than two regular friends
	More anxious and less sociable (teacher reports)
Neuropsychological	Speech difficulties (three times the normal rate) before age 15
	Later onset of walking
	Below-average educational test scores
Family	Difficulties in parenting/understanding (mother's reports)
	Different from other children (mother's reports)

3.32 Can one get schizophrenia as a child or a teenager?

Schizophrenia is rare before the late teens, but earlier-onset cases have been recognized. These include the so-called 'disintegrative psychoses of childhood', 'propf-schizophrenia' and straightforward, very-early-onset schizophrenia in early teenagers. The former are rare and are often associated with brain disorders and early dementia. Propf-schizophrenia is the combination of an established learning difficulty (formerly known as mental handicap) with schizophrenia-like symptoms, it being difficult to establish which came first. Early teenage schizophrenias are no different from ones of older onset but, because of immaturity and hormonal changes, can be hard to distinguish from mood disorders. Symptoms are often non-specific, such as declining school grades, difficulty interacting with others, vague complaints of teasing or physical symptoms and even a degree of self-neglect. Unfortunately, the earlier the onset, the worse the prognosis, hence the importance of early diagnosis and treatment.

3.33 Can school problems be caused by schizophrenia?

Most children who find it difficult to cope with school, either not attending or being disruptive in class, certainly do not have a schizophrenic or pre-schizophrenic illness. The two most typical groups are children with school phobia and those with school avoidance (truanting). The former tend to have anxiety-based conditions (and often very anxious mothers) but once in school do quite well. The latter often come from disorganized and deprived home backgrounds, do not do well in class even when they are there (mild learning difficulties and/or conduct disorder being common bases) and require separate approaches. Looking back at the school careers of those who have subsequently developed schizophrenia, however, they will often have been referred to child guidance, they will have found it difficult to socialize (*see Q. 3.31*), and there may well be evidence of a decline in school performance. Clarifying such diagnoses in school-age children is, however, a specialist skill, and an early referral to the child psychiatrist is to be recommended.

 PATIENT QUESTIONS

3.34 If I hear voices, does that mean I must have schizophrenia?

No. Although hearing voices is the typical schizophrenic symptom, occurring in up to 70% or more of patients at some time in their illness, there are many other causes of 'hearing voices'. These include drugs (e.g. amphetamines and LSD), head injuries, ear disorders (e.g. tinnitus) and other forms of psychiatric illness. Voices can thus accompany some people when they are feeling very high or low (manic depressive illness) and can occur in states of great physical exhaustion or isolation (e.g. round-the-world yachtsmen).

The most common experience of 'normal' voices occurs when going off to or waking from sleep. It is reckoned that up to a quarter of people have had some kind of 'voice-like' experience, usually when they are half-awake. Voices heard when going off to sleep are called hypnagogic hallucinations, and those on waking hypnopompic hallucinations. They probably derive from bits of the brain falling asleep (or waking up) at a slightly different rate so a dream seems real or other noises get muddled up as a voice. Such experiences probably explain a belief in ghosts and other such phenomena.

3.35 Is it common to feel depressed even though you have schizophrenia?

Yes. Depression is unfortunately quite common in people who have schizophrenia, as in the population at large (up to 20%), and is often missed. This is because there tends to be an overlap of symptoms, and complaints of depression can be all put down to the voices or side-effects of medication. Studies show that about 7% of patients with schizophrenia have regular suicidal thoughts, whereas 10% or more sadly commit suicide. It is also not uncommon for people to feel depressed, that is to say unhappy, troubled, anxious and finding it hard to think, at the start of a schizophrenic illness or relapse. Recognizing these symptoms can be very useful in getting treatment early.

Becoming depressed, particularly when one has continuing schizophrenic symptoms (e.g. chronic voices) despite treatment, is also well recognized. This may be made worse by medication, particularly if it slows one down, by the embarrassment and stigma of having the illness (and sometimes by the attitudes of others) and by difficulties in thinking and concentrating.

The causes of schizophrenia

4

4.1   Do we know the cause of schizophrenia?

Despite extensive research no single, defined cause has been established, nor is the pathogenesis yet clarified. Based on the increasing evidence of subtle brain abnormalities, a significant genetic loading and an association with potentially traumatic events (e.g. obstetric complications and viral infections in utero), schizophrenia is currently viewed as a *neurodevelopmental* disorder. As a result of this combination of inherited and environmental factors, symptoms emerge towards the later stages of brain development, that is to say in adolescence or relatively soon after. Although some individual patients show a specific abnormality or lesion (e.g. a local head injury to the temporal lobe), the particular cause of an individual's illness can rarely be clarified.

4.2   How strong is the evidence for schizophrenia being an inherited disease?

It is now accepted that up to 70% or more of the risk for schizophrenia derives from genetic factors.[6] Not only are there a number of other genetic disorders associated with psychosis (e.g. Huntington's disease and porphyria), but the results of family, twin and adoption studies over a number of years have also increasingly shown the importance of inheritance. In fact, the observation that the illness runs in families was acknowledged by researchers before the First World War. The higher the genetic loading, the more likely one is to develop schizophrenia. Therefore, having an identical (monozygotic) twin who has schizophrenia, or two parents with schizophrenia, gives a 50% or more chance of developing the condition (*Fig. 4.1*).

4.3   Does schizophrenia always run in families?

No. Although genetic factors do play a significant part, inheritance is not transmitted in a true Mendelian fashion. Some patients certainly seem to have no family history, even several generations back, of psychotic illnesses, and the notion of a gene mutation or particular cerebral insult has to be considered. Current genetic theories are therefore relatively complex (and difficult to disprove or prove), but it is believed that there has to be an inheritance of a number of genes, interacting with each other and with environmental effects, to put a person 'over the top' in terms of developing the illness (*see also Case vignette 4.1*). This would also explain why many identical twins do *not* seem to share illnesses, although conditions such as

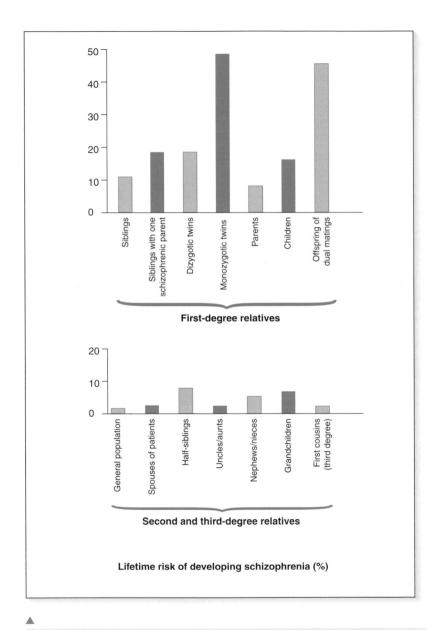

Fig. 4.1 Lifetime risk of developing schizophrenia. Data from twin studies of European populations, 1920–87

TABLE 4.1 Lifetime expectancy of broadly defined schizophrenia in the relatives of schizophrenics. Table reproduced with permission from Kendell R E, Zealley A K. *Companion to Psychiatric Studies*. Edinburgh: Churchill Livingstone, 1993

Relationship	Percentage schizophrenic
Parent	5.6
Sibling	10.1
Sibling and one parent affected	16.7
Children of one affected parent	12.8
Children of two affected parents	46.3
Uncles/aunts/nephews/nieces	2.8
Grandchildren	3.7
Unrelated	0.86

delusional disorder, schizotypal disorder and major depression are found more often than would be expected in the families of patients with schizophrenia. *Table 4.1* shows relatives' lifetime expectancy of developing schizophrenia.

CASE VIGNETTE 4.1

Alice and her younger brother John, aged 42 and 38 respectively, had both suffered from schizophrenia from their early 20s. Initially, they had been in and out of hospital for years despite a good response to standard antipsychotic treatments, including depot medication. They also received active outreach from a community nurse team, with whom they got on well, and attended a local day unit intermittently. The main factor preventing their continuing with treatment was that their mother (a widow) denied that they were ill and was very verbally aggressive, as well as sometimes physically threatening, to the community nurses. Furthermore, there were two older siblings who were also very critical about both the behaviour of their younger sister and brother, and those nurses whom they deemed to be 'causing the trouble'. They could not understand, for example, why Alice could not just 'pull herself together, get a job and get married'.

The family home was in a poor state, with holes in the roof (where pigeons were nesting) and a generally rather deteriorated air. After Alice and John had been ill for over 10 years, their mother died, and their older sister moved away to get married. Because of the nature of the house, which was now deemed unsafe, it became necessary to move the family to new accommodation. At this juncture, a nurse and a psychologist began to work regularly with the family, looking at the nature of the illness and using family psycho-education techniques. The two 'well' siblings became much more accepting of their younger sister's and brother's illnesses and allowed continued treatment to maintain them more properly in the community. John began attending a rehabilitation centre on a regular basis, improved benefits were obtained for both of them, and hospital admissions ceased. The use of a home care worker enabled both of them to live independently, with some support from their brother and sister, and they have had no relapses for over 10 years.

It was interesting that their long-'missing' father had in fact died in a mental hospital after a protracted (probably schizophrenic) illness.

4.4 Can schizophrenia be caused by child sexual abuse?

There is currently no evidence of a direct relationship between a psychotic illness, such as schizophrenia, and established sexual abuse in childhood. Although the latter condition has been shown, in several research studies, to reveal brain scan abnormalities, these do not seem to be especially associated with those reported in patients with schizophrenia. Individual patients may of course have experienced both conditions, as well as physical abuse (e.g. regular blows to the head) and possible nutritional neglect, which one could surmise to be associated with the kind of parents who would perpetrate child sexual abuse. Currently, no specific psychiatric condition can be definitively linked to such problems in childhood.

4.5 Are there any particular injuries or illnesses, in birth or early childhood, that are commonly associated with schizophrenia?

There are some established associations in the perinatal period that are, for reasons as yet unclear, considered to be significant risk factors. These include obstetric complications, patients with schizophrenia seeming to have more obstetric problems (e.g. a lower Apgar score), with probably a fourfold increase in risk, than controls. Intrauterine conditions, such as a viral infection, poor nutrition or rhesus incompatibility, also seem to increase risk, as do perinatal or early childhood head injuries and, to a much lesser degree, being born during the winter. The greatest increase in risk is associated with childhood encephalitis, now fortunately a relatively rare condition. See *Figure 4.2* for the relationship between obstetric complications and risk of schizophrenia.

4.6 Could schizophrenia be an infectious disease?

It certainly could, and there are alluring indications, both historical and associated with more recent research, pointing to this possibility.[7] The leading American psychiatrist E. Fuller Torrey, in his book *Schizophrenia and Civilisation*,[8] even suggested that the crowded industrial cities of the 19th century had created an infective agent that brought on an almost 'new' disease. The widespread prevalence of encephalitis lethargica (to some degree, possibly, a consequence of the 1918–20 influenza epidemic) led to a number of patients developing schizophrenic (especially catatonic) symptoms. Also the slight increase in winter birth rate – possibly associated with viral infections – and some evidence that a higher rate of schizophrenia is found in those who were in utero during influenza epidemics strengthen this association. In Russia, an increased rate of schizophrenia among residents of blocks of flats in whom one

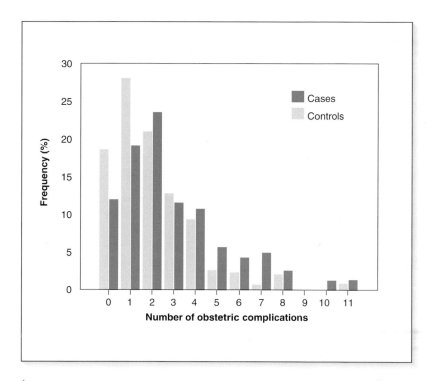

Fig. 4.2 The relationship between obstetric complications and risk of schizophrenia. Complications are more common in people with schizophrenia compared with controls, especially multiple complications. From Stefan M, Travis M, Murray R M 2002 *An Atlas of Schizophrenia.* Parthenon, London, with permission

schizophrenic patient has been living have also been reported (although this has not been confirmed by further research). However, direct studies of blood and cerebrospinal fluid, looking for raised antibody or antiviral titres in patients with schizophrenia, have so far proved negative.

4.7 Does smoking cannabis cause schizophrenia?

This is currently a most controversial topic, many researchers (and families) considering the relationship to be significant. However, in those countries in which cannabis smoking has been endemic over many years, there is no evidence of an increased rate of schizophrenia. The wonderfully named British Hemp Commission (a late Victorian study) likewise did not consider that hemp (i.e. cannabis) was causative, even though it was widely used by contemporary populations in India and Egypt.

On the other hand, a large-scale study of Swedish army recruits found that those admitting at recruitment to using or having used cannabis (particularly on a more than routine basis) had a sixfold risk of developing schizophrenia compared with non-users (*Fig. 4.3*).[9] Could this be seen as causative, or could it simply be that cannabis usage was a 'marker' of young men already experiencing the anxieties and uncertainties of impaired neurodevelopment? There is also the possibility that cannabis usage, particularly on a chronic level, may generate a pseudo-schizophrenic state in terms of paranoid ideation and lack of drive (so-called 'amotivational syndrome') in susceptible individuals (*see Q. 3.17*). The cannabis debate is summarized in *Table 4.2*.

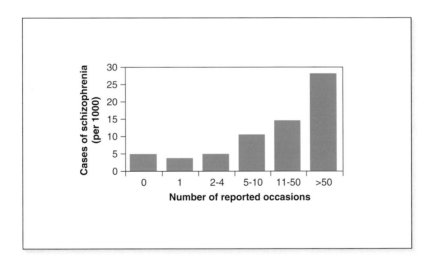

Fig. 4.3 Cannabis consumption at age 18 and later risk of schizophrenia. From Stefan M, Travis M, Murray R M 2002 *An Atlas of Schizophrenia*. Parthenon, London, with permission

4.8 Might any illicit drugs bring on schizophrenia?

Although many drugs (*see Table 3.6*) are associated with causing psychotic reactions, it is not clear whether they actually cause the onset of a genuine

TABLE 4.2 Does cannabis cause schizophrenia?	
For	**Against**
Can enhance 'paranoid' feelings and thoughts	Many patients find cannabis relaxes them
Increased cannabis use is associated with an increased risk of developing schizophrenia	There is no increased prevalence of schizophrenia in cannabis-using cultures
An increased incidence of schizophrenia has recently been reported (inner London)	Cannabis use is now widespread, but (comparatively) very few people have schizophrenia
Schizophrenic symptoms are worsened by cannabis use	Victorian doctors used cannabis to treat 'mania' (i.e. psychosis)

schizophrenic illness. Amphetamines ('speed') are particularly associated with developing an almost 'model' psychosis, characterized by paranoid delusions, hallucinations and even thought disorder or catatonia. Likewise, lysergic acid diethylamide (LSD), ecstasy (MDMA), cocaine, ketamine and mescaline are all associated with acute illnesses that are often indistinguishable from schizophrenia. Such drug-induced states are part of the routine differential diagnosis and generally resolve within several days.

There is, however, evidence from studies of LSD-induced psychosis that such patients, compared with other schizophrenia sufferers, have an onset 3 or 4 years earlier. It thus seems that LSD accelerates the onset of an illness that would probably have emerged anyway. Any unusual psychosis-like symptoms reported by those taking illicit drugs (and users will often be quite frightened by them) should lead to very firm advice to abstain forthwith because of these risks.

4.9   Is there any particular pattern of family dynamics or behaviour that seems to bring on schizophrenia?

Although there was, in the 1960s and 70s, a vogue for considering family behaviour as the key aetiology behind schizophrenia (as evidenced in the notorious 1971 film *Family Life*), the evidence for this has now largely been discredited. Particular notions included the 'double bind', whereby children were given conflicting messages by their parent (e.g. 'I love you very much but please leave the room'), and the theory of a 'schizophrenogenic mother'. Researchers claimed to be able to pick out such people via structured interviews, but apart from tending to talk more, no formal difference was subsequently found. Evidence from adoption studies, comparing the biological children of schizophrenic mothers with controls (also adopted but from healthy mothers), showed that biological parentage was the key factor (*see Q. 4.12*).

There is, however, good evidence that *relapse* can be enhanced by family style, those families showing high expressed emotion seeming to produce a worse relapse rate (*see Q 7.9* and *Box 7.1*).

4.10 Is schizophrenia a reaction to stressful or frightening life events?

Again, research in this area is not very clear, although there is limited evidence that the number of life events (i.e. events that are difficult to cope with, such as bereavement, job loss and moving house) do increase in the 3–6 months prior to the onset of the illness. However, because of the tendency of schizophrenia to have a fairly long prodromal stage, often months or even years, separating out cause and effect is quite difficult. Did the patient lose his job because he was getting unwell or vice versa? The effect is also much less than that for depressive illness, and there is a great variation in life events rather than just the experience of losses. Given our knowledge of the complex basis and course of schizophrenia, however, it would not be surprising if such individuals were vulnerable to psychological stress.

4.11 Is schizophrenia commoner in poorer families?

Not necessarily, although the effect of schizophrenic symptoms is very much to promote a degree of social decline. Studies have thus shown that, using social class as a criterion, the fathers of patients with schizophrenia ranged right across the social spectrum in the proportions one would expect. In many cases, therefore, the patients themselves will unfortunately slide down the social scale and will present as being in poorer social circumstances. This probably accounts for the long-standing finding, deriving from social research in Chicago in the 1930s, that inner city areas tend to have a higher rate of schizophrenia – because of the cheaper lodging houses or hostels available in these areas. Similar considerations apply to impoverished rural areas, for example parts of Ireland, more active and enterprising souls emigrating for economic reasons.

Because the genetics of schizophrenia are non-Mendelian, it does not necessarily follow that the children of schizophrenic patients will have schizophrenia – in fact, about 90% will not. There is thus no overall clustering effect towards poorer families as non-affected children will have an equal chance to go up or down the social scale. This process has been termed 'social drift', rather than a 'social shift' (as one would expect were the inheritance more straightforward), but there are arguments for and against this belief, and very recent research suggests that city life seems to 'encourage' schizophrenia.

4.12 Does the way in which individuals are brought up make it more or less likely that they will develop schizophrenia (*see also Q. 4.9*)?

There is no evidence that any particular style of parenting makes it more or less likely for someone to develop an illness such as schizophrenia. Various adoption studies have shown that the key factor is one's biological parentage rather than parenting style. Thus, children adopted away from their mothers have been followed up to see how many would develop schizophrenia. Some of these children had mothers with schizophrenia; others came from 'normal' families. One would expect a similar outcome in those with a similar family upbringing, but schizophrenia was in fact much commoner in those with a (biological) schizophrenic mother. Thus, although a stable upbringing is clearly related to one's personality style, ability to cope with stress and some forms of depression, and although schizophrenia is not just genetic in origin, upbringing in itself does not seem to be significant in causation.

4.13 Does your school have any effect on whether you will get schizophrenia?

There is no evidence that the school environment will promote or protect individuals from schizophrenia (*see also* Q. 3.32 and 3.33). There is evidence that schoolchildren who go on to get schizophrenia show some behavioural abnormalities, such as increased social anxiety, some difficulties in learning and a tendency to make few friendships, but often such anomalies are only seen as significant when reviewed after the child has developed the illness. There have been no studies on whether symptoms are potentially enhanced by the consequent experiences of troubled children at school (e.g. teasing and teachers' exasperation), but, given the known environmental sensitivity of patients with schizophrenia, more research is required. It would, on the face of it, seem sensible to have an appropriate awareness of such presentations so that early assessment and referral, by educational psychologists and child psychiatrists, can be made if necessary.

4.14 Is schizophrenia due to a chemical imbalance in the brain?

Almost certainly yes. The dominant theory, until the 1990s, was based around dopamine. This was derived from the known effects of dopamine-blocking drugs in successfully counteracting some schizophrenic symptoms, and the contrary symptom-inducing effects of dopaminergic drugs (e.g. antiparkinsonian agents). The phenomenon of catalepsy (unusual posturing and muscle tone) in rats given such agents further supported the theory. Repeated attempts to develop a blood test for schizophrenia have, however, so far failed.

The development of 'atypical' antipsychotics has more recently led to a more refined theory based around an imbalance between dopamine and serotonin (also known as 5-hydroxytryptamine or 5HT). In particular, atypical drugs such as clozapine block 5HT at certain receptor sites, whereas hallucinogenic drugs such as mescaline and LSD are very much 5HT agonists. It may be that blocking 5HT has an indirect effect on dopamine pathways, but the exact details require further research. Other theories relate to neurotransmitters such as acetyl choline and glutamate, and it may well be that different symptoms are related to different neurochemical abnormalities.

4.15 Is schizophrenia associated with any other illnesses in particular?

Associations with schizophrenia, in terms of other physical illnesses, are few and far between, largely deriving from the consequences of having schizophrenia in the first place. Thus, the tendencies to smoke excessively, to take little exercise and to have poor dietary habits seems to lead to a higher incidence of conditions such as bronchitis, heart disease and type 2 diabetes mellitus. The effects of medication, whether traditional or atypical antipsychotics, tend to enhance this, particularly in terms of weight gain. There is, however, evidence that there is anyway a higher rate of diabetes and 'pre-diabetes' (i.e. abnormal glucose tolerance) – of the order of 10% or more – in patients with schizophrenia. This will of course be exacerbated by weight gain, and routine blood sugar monitoring can be important in treatment.

The association between deafness and late-onset schizophrenia is stronger. Up to a third of these older patients will have some degree of hearing impairment, and there are also higher rates – up to 10% or more – of schizophrenic and delusional illnesses in patients with primary hearing impairment. It has been posited that the social isolation of deafness or some degree of hearing impairment may enhance delusional ideation. Alternatively, some underlying temporal lobe abnormality may be a factor in generating the impaired neural functioning associated with deafness in patients who already have schizophrenia.

4.16 Has modern research enhanced our understanding of how schizophrenia is caused?

Modern theories of the causation of schizophrenia are centred around the notion of a 'neurodevelopmental' disorder. Thus, given the strong genetic basis, it is assumed that one inherits a genetic abnormality, which is acted upon via a variety of risk factors. These include obstetric problems, infections (e.g. rubella or even influenza), and any kind of brain damage or infection in early infancy. It is suggested that this combination of genetic vulnerability and subtle forms of brain impairment leads over time to an illness that only expresses itself when the brain is fully matured (*Fig. 4.4*).

The unusual rate of minor brain abnormalities (e.g. on computed tomography scans), the cognitive and behavioural oddities in children, and the increased rate of minor physical anomalies all support this theory. Overall, it is suggested that about 30% of the risk of schizophrenia is therefore related to these various factors, so there may be an association between improved obstetric care and current theories of a small decline in the incidence of schizophrenia, at least in developed countries.

4.17 Is schizophrenia just a reaction to the pressures of modern life?

No. Although there is evidence that patients with schizophrenia have experienced significant life events in the period prior to their illness, it is difficult to distinguish cause from effect. It may be, for example, that their reaction to a life event is unusual in itself, which is important given the ups

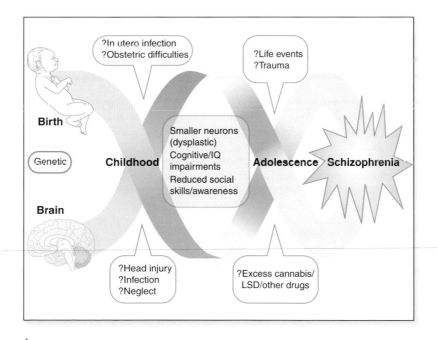

Fig. 4.4 Causality over the life course. Risk factors for schizophrenia occur both early and late in the life course, and interact with each other in a complex fashion

and downs of life, particularly the pressures and changes that take place in the lives of younger people. The death of a parent may, for example, lead to a bereavement reaction that creates a psychotic breakdown (such as schizophrenia) in a vulnerable individual. On the other hand, it may be that the parent was in fact protecting someone who was already ill so the illness comes to light only once the parent is no longer around.

There is no evidence that specific aspects of modern life, such as diet, high-speed travel, atmospheric pollutants or the hurly-burly of numerous information sources (e.g. television and mobile phones) are in any sense causative of the illness. Difficulties in coping with the faster pace of life, particularly in urban environments, may of course be highly involved in creating problems for patients with schizophrenia. There is thus some evidence of an improved prognosis in Third World countries, particularly in agrarian environments, which is intriguing and worthy of continuing research.

4.18 Is there anything in particular that can be done to prevent schizophrenia developing?

Given the tendency to genetic loading, with possible obstetric risk factors, any preventative programme would have to address these rather difficult issues. Identifying the relevant gene (or set of genes) could in time make for prenatal diagnosis, as has occurred, for example, with Down's syndrome, while discouraging people with schizophrenia from marrying and having children could theoretically also be tried. Such eugenic approaches do of course have a rather unpleasant history. Improved obstetric care (*see* Q. 4.16) should also be of benefit, given the known higher rate of obstetric complications. The prevention of childhood (as well as prenatal) infections may also be of some help, but there is currently no evidence that the viral vaccination programme has led to any significant change in the incidence of schizophrenia. Current research is also focusing on potential 'pre-schizophrenic' children, giving them antipsychotic medications (and even cognitive therapy) prior to the overt (likely) onset of their illness, in order to prevent its active expression.

4.19 Are there any genetic tests for schizophrenia?

There are currently no specific genetic tests for schizophrenia, although a number of specific genes in large family aggregations have been isolated. Unlike Mendelian-dominant conditions, such as Huntington's chorea, it is not possible at present to provide any definitive tests. Although certain chromosomes have been targeted because of particular findings (e.g. chromosome 5, and chromosome 22 because of its association with the unusual developmental disorder velocardiofacial syndrome), again nothing definite has been established. As the mode of inheritance is unclear, such approaches will continue to run into considerable difficulties in terms of searching for a specific gene. Nevertheless, genetics is clearly part of the key to the mystery, interacting with environmental factors to create increased risks of illness (*Fig. 4.5*).

4.20 Can schizophrenia be brought on or worsened by the constituents of one's diet?

There is no evidence that different diets can enhance or trigger schizophrenic symptoms. There have been a number of theories surrounding vitamin consumption, and fears that there may be an association with the allergies associated with milk or gluten. However, the vitamin story derives largely from studies of pellagra, a vitamin deficiency syndrome associated with lack of niacin in the diet. Pellagra can present with a range of psychological abnormalities, apparently including schizophrenia-like symptoms such as hallucinations, as well as skin and bowel problems. The converse, that other forms of vitamin deficiency (e.g. of vitamin C or D) must therefore be involved in schizophrenia, is *not true*. Serious deficiency diseases, for example of vitamin B12, can of course have wide-ranging effects including psychological symptoms, although these are

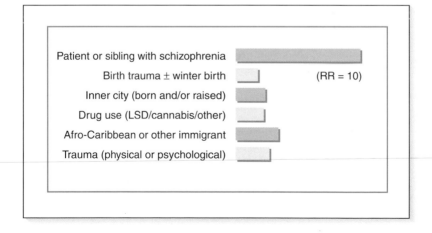

Fig. 4.5 Risk factors and effect sizes. There is no single cause of schizophrenia. Instead, like other complex disorders such as coronary heart disease, a number of genetic and environmental factors interact to cause the disease

usually neuropsychiatric, for example Wernicke–Korsakoff syndrome secondary to thiamine deficiency.

4.21 Is schizophrenia commoner in inner city areas?

Almost certainly yes. There are a number of reasons for this, generally associated with the 'drift' hypothesis, suggesting that the impairments of schizophrenia lead to people sliding down the social scale. Cheap flats, hostels and inner city lodgings therefore tend to have a greater schizophrenic population. Other researchers have suggested that a poor early environment (leading to infections or complications during the perinatal period) is associated with impoverished families who are more likely to live in deprived, over-crowded inner city areas, so that inner cities breed their own enhanced number of schizophrenics. Overall, it is probable that both of these factors account for the increased rate of schizophrenia in inner city areas, and the changes in the property market (inner city London being now increasingly expensive) may in time help to throw light on this problem. Schizophrenia is also more *apparent* in big cities, for example downtown Chicago or New York, simply because of the sheer number of cases involved. (*See Case vignette 4.2.*)

CASE VIGNETTE 4.2

A 25-year-old woman, unknown to the psychiatric services, was reported by her landlord because of concerns about her being a fire risk. She had moved to inner London from Oxford some 5 months previously and seemed to have no particular contacts with people locally. She had consulted a local GP for headaches and, it emerged, also threatened the landlord with legal action because of what she deemed to be his 'interference' in her day-to-day activities. A home visit was arranged, and the lady agreed to be interviewed, standing in the kitchen of her somewhat decrepit flat.

There was very little in the way of furniture or belongings, there were matches all over the floor, and there were no signs of food anywhere. During the interview the patient, who was oddly dressed in a long black gown (but nothing else), drank from a glass of wine, which she also threw over the assessing psychiatrist when she became annoyed. She was wearing no shoes, had oddly bleached hair and emitted a slightly unpleasant body odour. She was unwilling to describe the reasons for her actions but merely insisted that there had been a deliberate orchestration of the visit, although she would not elaborate on the agency, whom she hinted at controlling what was going on. She admitted to being under 'continual observation' and being 'prevented from working', insisting also that the visiting doctor and social worker had been ordered 'what to wear'. Her mood came across as irritable and hostile, and the nature of her ideas (when further explored) clearly amounted to a complex paranoid delusional system.

Recommendations were made for her detention under the Mental Health Act and it subsequently emerged that she had in fact had two previous admissions in her home town and had run away from her biological mother, who also had a long-term mental illness.

4.22 Could schizophrenia be caused by toxic chemicals or other pollutants?

Although there have been a number of local outbreaks of toxic chemicals, for example at Camelford in Cornwall (aluminium) and Minemata in Japan (mercury), none of these has been associated with an increase in the rate of schizophrenia. The usual cerebral reaction leads to forms of dementia or other cognitive impairments. Nor has there been shown to be any association between schizophrenia and particular geographical areas, for example near to nuclear power plants or other sites of industrial pollution. This does not of course exclude the possibility that vulnerable individuals might be affected by certain toxins, but the neuropathological findings in schizophrenia do not show that any specific reaction has taken place.

4.23 What are the chances of us knowing more about the causes of schizophrenia in the near future?

Research into genetics, brain-scanning and new forms of antipsychotic drugs could well lead to advances in our understanding of the aetiology of this condition. Establishing the chromosomal basis, for example of people with definite schizophrenia, would enable a clearer picture of the pathophysiology. Being able to isolate particular 'hot spots' in the brain, via sophisticated probes, could likewise point to clear neurochemical or neuropathological abnormalities. The development of newer (atypical) drugs, as with the development of dopamine-blocking agents in the 1950s, has already enhanced our understanding of a possible biochemical basis. What is clear is that the evidence accumulating on the causes of schizophrenia points to a significant form of cerebral disorder (*Table 4.3*).

4.24 Is schizophrenia equally common in other countries?

All the evidence shows that the prevalence of schizophrenia is roughly the same around the world. This applies to industrialized as well as developing countries and equatorial regions as well as countries in higher latitudes. In this sense, schizophrenia lies in particular contrast to disorders such as multiple sclerosis, which has clear latitudinal differences. Although there are some reported emigration effects (*see Q. 3.23*), this consistent prevalence seems to point to a somewhat unique basis for the disease. It may well be, for example, a natural consequence of evolution, the genetic mutation that enabled *Homo sapiens* to develop an enlarged forebrain (and thus an extraordinary range of skills such as speech and memory), perhaps bringing with it a risk potential for a small proportion of the population.

TABLE 4.3 The aetiology of schizophrenia – likely research approaches

Technique	Application
Brain scans (positron emission tomography/magnetic resonance imaging)	Localizing the abnormality Linking symptoms to brain areas
Genetics Establishing robust sites of chromosomal abnormalities	Establishing pattern of inheritance Determining how much of the risk is inherited
Neurochemistry	Abnormalities in specific neurochemicals, e.g. dopamine and noradrenaline
Receptor abnormalities or changes in specific brain areas	Effects of drugs (medical or illicit) on specific neurochemical activity
Psychosocial	Epidemiology of prevalence/incidence in given populations Effects of stress factors (family, trauma, culture) on vulnerable individuals

The main difference in terms of the public face of schizophrenia in different countries is the attitude towards the illness. Social stigma leads many families (e.g. in India or Japan) to keep their relatives out of the public eye, whereas in the USA it is quite common to see obviously psychotic 'street people' wandering around talking to themselves in downtown areas. It is also likely that, in the impoverished metropolises of the Third World, the life expectancy of seriously disordered people is very low, hence the apparent variations in numbers reported.

4.25 Is schizophrenia commoner in creative people or scientists?

There is no evidence available to answer this. Although schizophrenia has been associated with creativity, for example the obvious similarities between a delusion (i.e. a new but false belief) and a 'brainwave', the impairments of the illness tend to militate against high-powered achievement. There have nevertheless been certain famous cases of people who have had the illness; the ballet dancer Nijinski, for example, and the American mathematician portrayed in the recent film *A Beautiful Mind*. It is sometimes stated that schizoid characteristics are advantageous for people who are involved with test-tubes or computers, but these personality traits need to be differentiated from the full-blown illness. There is some evidence that bipolar affective disorder (manic depressive illness) is more common among writers and artists, but the same does not seem to be true of schizophrenia.

4.26 Does schizophrenia carry any evolutionary advantage?

It probably does. If one takes the core symptoms of schizophrenia, namely hallucinations, delusions, passivity experience and forms of thought disorder or interference, one can see them as faulty versions of highly developed evolutionary skills. Thus, the ability to create new ideas, the ability to connect up thoughts and develop memories, the ability to put together a wide range of perceptual inputs in order to appreciate one's environment, and the ability to know what is you and what is not you can all be seen as vital and advantageous skills. Even obviously distressing experiences, for example paranoid beliefs that people are following you, could be seen as advantageous in a hostile environment. Being over-sensitive (rather than easily surprised) to threats, or even misinterpreting non-specific noise as the approaching footsteps of a predator, should, all in all, enhance life expectancy.

 PATIENT QUESTIONS

4.27 Can schizophrenia be passed on like an infection, for example by touching or kissing someone?

There is no evidence at all that schizophrenia is transmitted like an infection. Partners and parents, who often share houses, cutlery, food and drink with those who have schizophrenia, do not 'catch' anything from them. There is of course an increased rate of schizophrenia among relatives, and the condition is well understood as an inherited phenomenon. Thus, although it is more likely, if you have schizophrenia, that one of your parents may have schizophrenia, they will have passed through the risk period by the time you develop the illness. There is also no increased risk at all for girlfriends or boyfriends, for example, nor can any kind of infection be passed on via sexual transmission. Schizophrenia is essentially an inherited illness, brought on or worsened by the subtle forms of brain damage that can happen variably in one's birth or early childhood. Affectionate physical contact is just as nice for schizophrenia sufferers as it is for anyone else.

4.28 If your brother or sister has schizophrenia, are you likely to pass it on to your children?

As outlined in *Figure 4.6* and *Table 4.1*, the relative risk of schizophrenia very much depends on how closely related you are to a sufferer. Thus, an identical twin has about a 50% risk, possibly more, a first-degree relative (parent, sibling or child) has about a 10% risk and a second-degree relative about a 3% risk. Second-degree relatives include uncles and aunts as well as nephews and nieces. The chance of a schizophrenic illness developing in one of your children if your brother or sister has schizophrenia is therefore

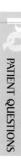

about 3 in 100. That is to say, 97 out of 100 of your (potential) children will *not* get the illness. Because the general prevalence of schizophrenia is about 1% (i.e. 99 out of 100 people do not have it), there is not a great deal of difference between the risk to your children and the risk to other children generally. If you are concerned about your family's risk, it is perfectly reasonable to consult your GP or a psychiatrist specializing in genetics. N.B. The information here refers to blood relatives and *not* relatives by marriage.

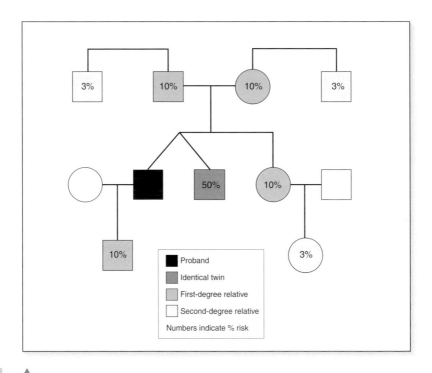

▲
Fig. 4.6 A genogram showing risk of schizophrenia in relatives. Adapted from Lewis, S, Buchanan, R W 1998 *Fast Facts Schizophrenia* Health Press Oxford, with permission

Psychiatric disorders with schizophrenia-like presentations

5.1   Are schizophrenic symptoms seen in other illnesses?

Yes. Whereas delusions and hallucinations, in particular, are seen as the hallmark of schizophrenia, they can in fact also appear as part of the presentation of other conditions. By contrast, formal thought disorder, passivity experience and negative symptoms (i.e. flat affect) are more specific to schizophrenia. Even so, it is always the combination of specific symptoms *and* the course of the illness *and* the exclusion of, for example, organic factors that clinches a true diagnosis of schizophrenia.

Practically speaking, hallucinations and delusions should be seen as almost non-specific indicators of brain malfunction, just as fever and an increased pulse rate are non-specific physical reactions to any number of illnesses. Thus, anyone can hallucinate if ill enough from brain damage, infection or physical deprivation, and visual hallucinations are the typical modality for organic disorders. Likewise, delusions, especially of grandeur, are common in manic illnesses and are of course the key element of delusional disorder (see below), in which they are the only symptom. The commonest basis for the incorrect diagnosis of schizophrenia lies in just these kinds of condition, in which a single psychotic symptom has been elicited but not enough attention has been paid to the overall pattern of presenting features (*see also Ch. 2*).

5.2   What is the commonest basis for schizophrenia being mistaken for another diagnosis?

There is little hard evidence on this, but some studies indicate the diagnoses patients receive before eventually being recognized as schizophrenic. The commonest of these is depression, some patients having several episodes of 'depression', which may even seem to respond to antidepressants, before the overt schizophrenic symptoms emerge. Likewise, manic episodes can very much resemble schizophrenia, particularly if there are grandiose delusions as well as some hallucinations, and the wise clinician awaits the outcome over several years before deciding which is which.

Although such mood disorders comprise the commonest mistake, cases of severe panic syndrome (and their rather paranoid and self-conscious fears of being out of doors) can also lead to mistaken diagnosis. Misuse of drugs, especially amphetamines and even cannabis in higher doses, can engender symptoms that mimic schizophrenia. A standard problem in psychiatry is differentiating the paranoid experiences of those who drink too much (or suddenly stop) or take drugs from the findings in those who use drugs or drink to suppress primary schizophrenic symptoms.

5.3 What are the typical symptoms of manic depressive (bipolar) psychosis?

These are outlined in *Table 5.1* and can readily be divided up into manic and depressive presentations. Manic patients often have grandiose delusions, believing, for example, that they have extra special abilities, are descended from royalty or have untold reserves of hidden wealth. Such beliefs, combined with a tendency to jump from topic to topic ('flight of ideas'), can sometimes be muddled with thought disorder. The presence of fleeting hallucinations can further confuse the picture.

Likewise, in depressive presentations, patients can have quite bizarre, 'nihilistic' delusions about their body being rotted away or even that they have no stomach or no blood in their veins. States of mutism and stupor are seen in both depression and schizophrenia, and clarification may sometimes be obtained only after treatment (e.g. with electroconvulsive therapy, or ECT) to find out the basis of such presentations. Delusions with a paranoid (persecutory) flavour can also occur, in either state, although so-called 'mood-congruent' delusions (i.e. negativity or over-the-top ideas) form the typical manic depressive presentation.

5.4 Can schizophrenic patients have manic symptoms?

It is often quite difficult to know whether someone who is psychotic, overactive, perhaps laughing a lot and claiming to have special powers has a schizophrenic or a manic illness. There are considerable overlaps in the presentation, and it is not uncommon for patients to be diagnosed as manic *and* schizophrenic on separate admissions. In addition, some forms of fatuity – the 'buffoonery syndrome' – can have a strongly manic feel, particularly if patients tend to talk on and on, semi-incoherently, laughing all the time and perhaps making others laugh too.

TABLE 5.1 **Symptoms of manic depressive (bipolar) psychoses**

Manic phase	Depressive phase
Irritable/euphoric mood	Depressed/suicidal mood
Flight of ideas	Psychomotor retardation
Pressure of speech	Incoherence or mutism
Grandiose delusions	Delusions of poverty/nihilism/guilt*
Hyperactivity	Stupor
Fleeting hallucinations	

*e.g. I've ruined the whole family; there's no blood in my body; I've committed unpardonable sins

Such overlap of symptoms often takes a succession of presentations to clarify, patients gradually moving towards one clear-cut diagnosis or the other. Unfortunately, it is an established pattern that manic or even depressive presentations tend to evolve into more obvious forms of schizophrenia over time. Statistical analysis – in the form of factor analysis – also shows that there is much greater overlap between manic and schizophrenic symptom patterns than a strict separation of the psychoses would justify, which is the basis for theories of a 'unitary psychosis'. That is to say, it is postulated that presentations of psychotic illness lie on a continuum of increasing severity, clearly manic or schizophrenic illnesses being merely two of the more obvious forms of presentation. The typical differences are summarized in *Table 5.2*.

5.5   Is it easy to mix up manic depressive and schizophrenic illnesses?

This certainly can occur, especially given the difficulty that can arise in distinguishing between depressive and negative symptoms. The limited speech, flattened affect, anhedonia (inability to enjoy things) and apathy that are part and parcel of negative symptoms can seem like the depressed mood, loss of concentration, tiredness and general slowing down that is the essence of depression. In addition, patients with depression can present with an obvious picture of slowing down – known as psychomotor retardation – which may resemble the semi-mute and stuporous states of catatonic schizophrenia. The convictions of severe depressives that they have carried out some dreadful deeds, or even, for example, that they are a witch who deserves to be burned at the stake, often have the bizarre quality of schizophrenic delusions.

TABLE 5.2 Some differences between manic and schizophrenic psychoses

	Mania	Schizophrenia
History	Acute onset with periods of stability	Persisting symptoms arising from a slower onset
Behaviour	Overactive/loud /'on the go'	Variable; fearful/agitated/'flat'
Symptoms	Predominant mood disorder	Mainly thought-disordered, hallucinated or delusional
Dress	Colourful, changeable	Shabby/bizarre; unchanging
Talk	Fast, detailed, loquacious, spontaneous	Often muddled, incoherent, limited
Family reaction	Exhausted but involved	Confused, disengaging

Research studies also seem to show that up to 20% or more of schizophrenics do seem to benefit from antidepressants – and seem to have depressive symptoms as well as negative symptoms – which complicates matters even more. The regular and close examination of an individual's mental state is most important in clarifying these uncertainties. A trial of treatment may sometimes be required on a best-guess basis.

5.6   What is meant by the terms 'acute' and 'reactive' psychosis?

Table 5.3 outlines a number of terms used to describe uncommon forms of illness that do not fit with either manic depressive or schizophrenic presentations, yet psychiatrists keep coming across them. There is a long history of such classifications, the 'reactive' or 'psychogenic' psychoses being especially popular in Scandinavia (apparently accounting for up to a fifth of all first-time admissions for psychosis in Denmark).[10] These essentially portray the onset of psychotic symptoms quite quickly (e.g. within several weeks) after a particular stressful event. It is also important that the content of the symptoms – that is to say the type of delusion – reflects the same traumatic event. Although patients can become quite seriously unwell, the diagnosis predicts full recovery, usually within 2–3 months (*Case vignette 5.1*).

Such brief psychoses have been the subject of enormous debate in the psychiatric world for many years. They are in some ways very similar to puerperal psychoses (*see Q. 5.7*) with their combination of psychotic symptoms, a degree of confusion and a rather changing picture. The *ICD-10* term is 'acute polymorphic psychosis', which reflects this rather chameleon-like pattern of presentation.[4]

CASE VIGNETTE 5.1 (ACUTE PSYCHOSIS)
A 45-year-old woman, working as a telephone operator, reported late for work. She had complained of flu-like symptoms for several days and found it difficult to

TABLE 5.3 Psychoses that are not schizophrenic and not manic depressive

	In DSM-IV	In ICD-10[4]	
Schizoaffective disorder	✓	✓	
Schizophreniform disorder	✓	–	
Psychogenic/reactive psychosis	–	–	acute
Brief psychotic disorder	✓	–	and
Acute polymorphic psychosis	–	✓	uncommon
Atypical/cycloid/periodical psychoses	–	–	severe
Bouffée délirante (France)	–	–	illnesses

settle down at her desk. She kept on getting up, seemed to be confused as to the time and beqan shouting down the phone at customers. Because of her behaviour, she was asked to leave the work area and was urgently assessed. She agreed to go to hospital but subsequently had to be detained because of increasingly paranoid beliefs about people trying to kill her, fuelled by auditory hallucinations and a belief that something had been implanted into her head. Her behaviour varied from the assaultative to the emotionally withdrawn, when she would be weeping with fear at her predicament.

All investigations, including an encephalogram (EEG) and computed tomography (CT) brain scan, proved negative, the lady responded over the course of 3 weeks to antipsychotic medication, and within 6 weeks of her initial breakdown she was coherent, no longer hallucinating, apologetic and appropriately behaved. She was continued on prophylactic antipsychotic medication for a number of months, on a gradually reducing dosage, went back to her work without problems and was medication-free within a year. Five years on, no further relapse had been reported.

5.7 What is a puerperal psychosis?

This is an acute psychotic illness that affects mothers within a week or two of giving birth to a child. Cases are rare, affecting about 1 in 500 of all births, but can affect up to 20% of subsequent births if the mother has already had an episode of puerperal psychosis. Although manic and paranoid symptoms are most common, some patients have very typical schizophrenia-like illnesses. Because of their variable presentation, they are classified separately from schizophrenia and bipolar disorders. Disorientation can be a particular feature, a mixed pattern of symptoms being not uncommon. Delusional beliefs that the child is imperfect or abnormal (or even evil), as well as suicide attempts, require careful assessment so admission to a Mother and Baby unit is usually vital. Most patients, unless this is the exacerbation of a pre-existing schizophrenic illness, recover fully within a month or two so treatment is very rewarding. A possible hormonal basis for these illnesses has been postulated, but no formal endocrine abnormality has been established.

5.8 Can people have both schizophrenic and manic depressive conditions at the same time?

The occurrence of such presentations is generally subsumed under the notion of 'schizoaffective psychoses' (*see* Q. 5.9); there is, however, a theoretical possibility of having both conditions (although this is very, very rare). It is thus possible for patients with schizophrenia to become much more agitated and overactive at times, or to become withdrawn and low. Distinguishing these reactions from the effects of medication, personal surroundings, or even the use of drugs can be very difficult.

5.9 What is meant by a 'schizoaffective' psychosis?

This is an unusual condition in which patients seem to have both affective (manic/depressive) and schizophrenic symptoms during the same episode of illness. Patients are sometimes described as 'schizomanic' or 'schizodepressive'. The details of these are outlined in *Table 5.4*. It needs to be stressed that both types of symptom must be present *at the same time* rather than just following each other at separate times, for example in different episodes of illness. Furthermore, this diagnosis should not be confused with the kind of depressive symptoms that come on after a psychotic illness such as schizophrenia (post-schizophrenic depression) or with the types of manic depressive illness that have delusions and hallucinations, giving them a schizophrenic 'feel'.

Some clinicians use the term 'schizoaffective psychosis' to describe an illness that has the course of manic depression, that is to say episodic illness followed by prolonged periods of remission, even though the dominant symptoms of illness (e.g. paranoid delusions) are more schizophrenic. It is just such confusions – and there are many in this field – that impair clarity of diagnosis. The general view is that such conditions are a kind of intermediate form of psychosis. They are not, however, particularly common, their frequency among psychiatric admissions being about 5%. It seems from genetic studies that schizomanic illnesses are quite closely related to manic conditions, whereas schizodepressive disorders are much more closely related to schizophrenia.

TABLE 5.4 Symptoms of schizoaffective disorders (as per *ICD-10*)[4]

Manic type	Depressive type
Elation ➔ grandiosity Excitement ➔ overactivity	Depressed mood ➔ retardation Hopeless ➔ suicidal Loss of energy, appetite, interest
With ■ Thought broadcast/interference ■ Hallucinations/passivity ■ Delusions (grandeur, persecution) **Overall picture**: Florid, acute onset, very disturbed behaviour but recovery within weeks (Sometimes also confused or even disorientated/perplexed)	*With* ■ Thought broadcast/interference ■ Threatening voices ■ Delusions (persecutory) **Overall picture**: Less florid than the manic type but tends to last longer. Most patients recover, but some later develop a more typical schizophrenia

5.10 What if people just have hallucinations and no other symptoms?

This is not common, but given the non-specific nature of hallucinations, as a symptom of many forms of brain disorder, it is not surprising that it occurs. Some people report hallucinations, usually a word or two, or a single image, on going off to sleep (hypnagogic) or on waking (hypnopompic), phenomena that seem to have a prevalence of some 20% in the overall population. Many patients cannot even be said to be unwell, whereas others have associated sleep or muscle tone disturbances such as narcolepsy or cataplexy (and more complex hallucinations). When there is no evidence of obvious mental illness, yet patients report what seem like abnormalities of hearing or sight, it is always important to check the hearing (e.g. tinnitus) and visual function (e.g. cataracts).

Some older people simply experience visual hallucinations, sometimes of small people or animals ('lilliputian hallucinations') and usually out of the corner of their eye. These may at times be quite vivid or distressing – although they can also be quite comforting – but they are not usually a schizophrenic symptom. Preserved intellect and insight, and clear consciousness (with or without eye pathology), has been named Charles Bonnet syndrome (after the French psychiatrist who first defined it), and is essentially harmless. By contrast, a constant or recurrent olfactory hallucination, for example the smell of burning rubber, is typically associated with temporal lobe epilepsy or even a temporal lobe tumour.

Pure auditory hallucinosis can also occur without any other obvious symptom or defect. Some chronic alcoholics develop a pure 'alcoholic hallucinosis' while they are drinking (as opposed to during withdrawal), and some individuals even develop musical hallucinations. Several famous mediums have relied on their chronic auditory hallucinations – and believed in them – as a form of communication with the spirit world. All of the above phenomena are, in their various forms, very much grist to the mill of those who believe in the supernatural or the paranormal (*see also Q. 1.15*).

5.11 If someone is deluded, does that usually mean they have schizophrenia?

Delusions (*see Q. 1.16*) are extremely common symptoms, typically associated with a psychosis such as schizophrenia but apparent in a number of conditions, probably as a non-specific response to both physical and psychological stressors. It is also important to separate out true delusions from what have been termed 'over-valued ideas', for example the attitude of anorexic girls towards their weight and body shape. Intense religious or even political beliefs seem at times to have a near-delusional quality, and these can shade into what has been termed 'delusional disorder' (*see Q. 5.13*).

Deciding whether someone whose only symptom is a delusion (or a number of delusions) has a schizophrenic illness will depend on the patient's age, social situation and intelligence. Bizarre beliefs, for example about aliens controlling one's mind or body, may merely be something of a metaphor in a gullible, perhaps not very bright, adolescent. More banal beliefs, for example an old lady convinced that the neighbours are mocking her or do not like her, may reflect a genuine social situation. Idiosyncratic cultural beliefs, for example Haitians believing in voodoo, may not fit with the formal criterion (of delusions) that they should not accord with one's sociocultural background. *Table 5.5* outlines some typical delusional presentations.

TABLE 5.5 Common types of delusion

Persecutory (common in delusional disorder)	Beliefs that one is being harassed, followed, interfered with, stolen from or threatened, by someone or some specific group, e.g. the IRA, the police, neighbours, people unknown, racists, etc.
Grandiose (often linked with manic psychoses)	Beliefs in one's own special powers or abilities to predict the future, affect world events or invent new devices or theories. Some patients may come to believe they are prophets, alien creatures or even Mohammed or Jesus Christ.
Of reference	Believing that television programmes, newspapers or various signals (e.g. traffic lights) or gestures (smiles or coughs) are specifically referring to oneself. Less intense 'ideas of reference' (i.e. non-delusional) are also common in both schizophrenia and panic states.
Of control (typically associated with passivity experience – see Table 2.1).	The sense that, for example, a computer or some other device or technical system is able to control oneself or others via various forms of ray, miasma, wiring or implantation.
Somatic	Beliefs that one's body is changed, deformed or even eaten away, or of an animal or 'devil' being inside one. May extend to nihilistic type (seen in severe depression) when one is convinced one has no stomach or intestines, or no blood in one's veins.
Relationships	Beliefs that a partner is having an affair (morbid jealousy), that an influential figure is secretly in love with you (erotomania) or that people are not really who they seem to be (e.g. Capgras syndrome).

5.12 What is folie à deux?

This rather evocative French phrase describes the way in which one person's psychotic beliefs can be imposed upon another. Thus, the more dominant partner in a married couple, or a parent with a rather impressionable son or daughter, can sometimes impose their delusions or even other psychotic experiences upon the weaker party. The non-psychotic partner may, for example, actually start believing that neighbours *are* bothering them, that voices *are* coming through the walls or that strange gases *are* being infused into their flat. The core illness (of the genuinely psychotic parent or spouse) may be a form of schizophrenia or a delusional disorder, with lack of insight as a key factor.

Diagnosis is, of course, made more difficult by the fact that the vital feature, namely a corroborative history, is lacking. The partner actually agrees with the (psychotic) patient that things really are being done to them. Community mental health or social work teams may spend weeks or even months looking for the cause of the harassment rather than locating the illness where it really is. The most important task is to separate the couple, within several days of which the 'weaker' partner will readily confess to having gone along with the symptoms they ascribed to.

Although folie à deux (i.e. only two people being involved) is the usual form, there can be a folie à trois or more (e.g. a whole family), or the effect can even take on a group form. Whether termed 'mass hysteria' or 'mass sociogenic illness', frightening outcomes have included the Jonestown massacre in Guyana and the sad events at Waco, Texas, USA, when the guru David Koresh persuaded his 'flock' to set fire to themselves rather than be intruded upon by United States law officers.

5.13 What is meant by the term 'delusional disorder'?

What used to be called 'paranoia' has now been renamed 'delusional disorder' in modern classifications such as *ICD-10*.[4] This is because the essence of this illness is the persistent and conspicuous presence of a long-held delusion or collection of delusions. In all other respects, the patients usually seem 'normal' in that their mood and how they speak, dress and behave is unexceptional. It is simply that they harbour, initially in a somewhat secretive fashion but as the disease goes on in a more disinhibited way, a particular delusional conviction. This may be a sense of persecution, for example that Freemasons are constantly interfering with their lives, or hypochondriacal, for example that they have a misshapen nose or head (particularly in younger age groups). It may of course also revolve around litigation or jealousy. The former ends up with patients being branded a 'querulous litigant' because they have so many actions before the court that the judges eventually decide they should be banned from such courses of action. Cases of 'morbid jealousy', with spouses being absolutely convinced that their partner is having an affair, can sadly lead to marital break-up, serious assault or even murder. The term 'Othello syndrome', from the Shakespearean tragedy depicting just such an outcome, is sometimes given to such cases. See *Box 5.1* for details of delusional disorders.

BOX 5.1 Delusional disorders (from ICD-10)[4]

This uncommon group of disorders (about 0.1% lifetime risk) used to be called 'paranoia' or even 'paranoid state' or 'paranoid psychosis'. There has been a constant debate amongst psychiatrists over how best to classify them.

Symptoms
A single delusion or a collection of delusional beliefs that forms a (usually complex) delusional system. These delusions increasingly dominate the patient's attitudes, relationships and behaviour. There are usually no other symptoms at all – i.e. no thought disorder, no self-neglect – thus the differentiation from schizophrenia (some older patients have occasional auditory or even tactile hallucinations, but only to a mild degree).

Onset and course
Usually in middle-aged (40–55 yrs) or older people. Somatic delusions (e.g. believing part of one's body is deformed) occur in younger folk. These illnesses generally tend to go on and on unrecognized, until quite severe and disabling, the patient becoming isolated, apparently embroiled in family or neighbour disputes, and seen by others as 'eccentric' or difficult.

Causes
Not known. Probably a combination of personality, life experiences and genetics, with possibly some brain insult triggering a gradual illness.

Clinical presentation
Patients often present only because of family insistence or legal necessities. Over several years (or even more) the delusional belief or system will have become dominant. Patients may be 'querulous litigants', taking out lawsuits because of a host of perceived slights or indignities. They may become hypochondriacal, convinced of a physical deformity or illness, seeking numerous assessments or even operations (e.g. 'delusional dysmorphophobia' leading to numerous cosmetic operations on one's face or body). Morbid jealousy, an unjustified conviction that one's partner is unfaithful, or erotomania, the conviction that someone else, often famous or influential, is in love with

them, can both lead to serious assaults or even murder. A general sense of persecution, by the police, racists, MI5 or the government, is another typical presentation (see the case vignette in the text). A secondary depression is, not surprisingly, quite common.

Treatment
This is often very difficult to initiate, the patient absolutely denying illness, let alone a 'mental' illness. Antipsychotics can be helpful, and cognitive approaches or problem-solving may be useful adjunctive therapies. Because of the non-compliance and self-isolation of many patients, evidence-based trials of treatment are, almost by definition, not available.

ASSOCIATED PHYSICAL DISORDERS

5.14 Are there any endocrine illnesses that can mimic schizophrenia?

The only condition recognized as doing this is hypothyroidism (myxoedema). Although hypothyroidism usually presents with obvious physical symptoms, for example dry skin, weight increase, slowed reflexes and voice changes, the development of paranoid delusions or even hallucinations in more severe cases is well known. This so-called 'myxoedema madness' is rarely seen today, given the availability of a biochemical diagnosis of thyroid disorders. By contrast, thyrotoxicosis does not produce such symptoms, although agitation and anxiety can dominate the clinical picture. Conditions such as Addison's disease and Cushing's syndrome are classic differential diagnoses of depression (or even mania with the latter case), whereas other endocrine disorders have no particular association with any mental illness. Pituitary tumours, if large, can of course be part of an organic psychosis, just like any other space-occupying brain lesion.

5.15 Are there any typical neurological or brain disorders that might have schizophrenic symptoms?

There are a number of such conditions, most of them not very common, but excluding them with simple tests and examinations is an important part of clarifying the diagnosis. The most important ones are outlined in *Table 3.4*, and it should be noted that the 'coarser' symptoms of delusions and hallucinations, often quite fleeting, are the usual psychiatric presentation. Subtler forms of schizophrenic symptomatology, such as thought broadcast or passivity experience, seem to be confined more to the true schizophrenia syndrome.

5.16 Can people with multiple sclerosis present with schizophrenic symptoms?

There is no evidence that schizophrenic illnesses or schizophreniform symptoms (i.e. individual symptoms rather than the whole illness) are more common in those with multiple sclerosis, but the prevalence of each illness (about 1%) makes it unsurprising that the two can coexist. Furthermore, given the brain lesions apparent, for example, on magnetic resonance imaging (MRI) scans of the brain, and given our current theories about the physical basis of schizophrenia, it should not be surprising that lesions of one condition (multiple sclerosis) could lead to symptoms of the other (schizophrenia). Psychotic states, if they do develop, usually come on around the time of the neurological abnormalities. Like all 'organic' psychoses, treatment is that much more difficult, and the use of steroids (e.g. to suppress the symptoms of multiple sclerosis) may of course even exacerbate any symptoms of schizophrenia.

5.17 Can epilepsy cause schizophrenia or vice versa?

There is a fascinating literature on the association between schizophrenia-like symptoms and epilepsy, either in the pre-ictal (before the fit) stage, during the fit or after it. This seems to be a specific condition, which has been heavily researched, that can benefit from both antipsychotics and anticonvulsants. There is, however, no evidence that epilepsy actually causes schizophrenia unless you have epileptic fits strongly related to the temporal lobe. In this sense, you will have a 'temporal lobe epilepsy' whereby the 'fits' may not comprise just falling down and shaking of the limbs, but may include hallucinations (visual, auditory and olfactory), an unusual sense of depersonalization or even strange, religious-like experiences.

In essence, epilepsy and schizophrenia do not cause each other despite the associated symptoms. Patients having unusual falls, faints, funny turns or blackouts in the context of ongoing schizophrenia-like symptoms should of course have an EEG. It should also be remembered that part of the theory for giving ECT to patients with schizophrenia (in the 1930s) was the notion that epilepsy excluded schizophrenia so fits would somehow be good for patients. Our current understanding points to a slight degree of overlap in terms of minor brain abnormalities on CT or MRI scanning, and an increased incidence of schizophrenic symptoms in patients with formal epilepsy, further enhancing the notion that schizophrenia is a form of brain disorder.

5.18 Is it easy to differentiate between late-onset schizophrenia and dementia?

There are usually clear differences in presentation between schizophrenia, whatever the patient's age, and dementia. The former condition will present with overt psychotic symptoms, and the older one is, the more likely these are to be just delusions and hallucinations. The more 'hebephrenic' symptoms of social decline, thought disorder and passivity are less apparent, although not unknown, in those over 50 years of age. By contrast, dementia presents with a gradual deterioration in intellectual function, including loss of memory, an impaired ability to carry out simple intellectual tests (e.g. subtracting serial sevens) and embarrassing behaviours reflecting this.

The dilemma arises when someone with, for example, Alzheimer's dementia first develops depressive or even paranoid symptoms (feeling people are out to harm them) of a vague nature that gradually evolve into more overt dementia. Regular, close observation of someone's cognitive state and checking how they cope with their day-to-day lives (can they find their way to the shops, can they remember to do basic tasks?) will soon clarify the diagnosis. This does not of course mean that treating the symptoms (e.g. giving antipsychotic agents for paranoid states) will not also be effective, at least in the early stages of the condition. Likewise, social decline and self-neglect in an elderly person, although usually caused by a dementia, may occasionally be a late form of schizophrenia. Admission will usually be needed to clarify matters.

5.19 Can schizophrenia cause a learning disability?

Because of symptoms such as muddled speech and social withdrawal, along with some old-fashioned equating of 'dementia praecox' with educational problems, there is considerable confusion over the case of schizophrenia as a disturbance of intellectual quotient (IQ). There are certainly similarities between people who are of impaired intelligence (learning disability) and those with schizophrenia in terms of their difficulties in school, their apparently 'childish' behaviours and their limited social skills, but the two conditions are distinctly different in terms of the diagnostic symptoms.

The key difference is that patients with a learning disability have been troubled by learning problems from early childhood onwards. They may well have had difficulties in walking and talking, or will have found it hard to cope with normal primary school; in terms of IQ testing (e.g. the Wechsler Adult Intelligence Scale) they do (by definition) have a formal impairment. By contrast, patients with schizophrenia may have reduced scores but nothing like as significant. They will have unusual ideas, thinking problems and a degree of social anxiety – they do not really like being in groups and find it hard to make friends – but this does not necessarily lead to an impaired IQ (the definition of a learning disability). There is some evidence that, with time, patients with schizophrenia do decline (e.g. by 5 or 10 points) in terms of their specific IQ score, but this usually takes 10–20 years. In a formal sense therefore, learning disability is something you are generally born with, whereas schizophrenia is an acquired change that can lead to a range of disabilities that may mimic learning problems.

ASSOCIATED SOCIAL PRESENTATIONS

5.20 Is it easy to 'pretend' to have schizophrenic symptoms?

The pretence of symptoms is much more difficult than it might seem to the sceptical lawyer or the hard-bitten physician. Claiming to have pretended such symptoms in itself has a poor prognosis, almost all patients ending up with long-term illnesses, of genuine severity, that often require continuing inpatient care. There was of course a famous experiment, carried out in the early 1970s, in which some psychology students presented themselves at hospitals in the USA claiming symptoms (e.g. a voice saying 'thud' in their ear).[2] All were accepted as inpatients, usually with a diagnosis of schizophrenia. This study has not been replicated, and it seems to have reflected the state of American psychiatry, particularly private psychiatry, in a certain epoch, rather vague, non-specific symptoms being part and parcel of what was deemed schizophrenia. Unless you have actually experienced the symptoms – and this is particularly obvious to a nurse or doctor with good clinical skills – it is extraordinarily difficult to go on acting out something like hearing a voice or believing in a delusion.

Part of the role of the acute psychiatric ward is to monitor and clarify just these uncertain presentations because there is a group of patients, whether they be deemed to have borderline personality disorders or simply to be difficult alcoholics, who insist they hear voices, voices telling them to do dreadful things, and insist that they must be admitted to hospital. Current risk management policies mean they have to be admitted because to do the alternative is, potentially, to ruin one's career. However, 2 or 3 days' observation by skilled nurses soon establishes the facts, while several simple tests (does the patient hallucinate in more than one modality, i.e. see *and* hear things at the same time? – because true schizophrenics do not) can help to clarify matters. When the condition is assessed by properly trained and experienced clinicians, schizophrenia remains extremely reliable as a formal diagnosis.

5.21 Do hysterical patients often present with schizophrenic symptoms?

No. The term 'hysteria' is now rather out of date, supposing as it does that people are pretending to have symptoms or are elaborating minor symptoms because of some kind of personality trait. The term 'hysteria' in fact derives from the Greek *husteros*, meaning the womb, and is based upon ancient notions of the womb rising or in other ways affecting one's psychological state. Such patients are now often deemed to have somatization disorders, or forms of anxiety, which can be diagnosed in terms of an appropriate mental state examination. Many complain of feeling faint, strange or even depersonalized (a sense of feeling unreal in yourself and things being unreal, like in a film, all around you), and they may even describe auditory hallucinations (albeit not in the third person) or a sense of their bodies being controlled (passivity). The differentiation between such states is clinically easy to clarify but often requires detailed mental state assessments as well as ongoing observation.

5.22 How do you differentiate between schizophrenia and personality disorder (*Table 5.6*)?

This can be difficult and remains one of the most important roles of an acute psychiatric unit as direct mental state assessment, for example in a GP's surgery, often cannot clarify such matters. In essence, patients with schizophrenia will have been well and will *then* have become ill, whereas those suffering from a 'personality disorder' will always have been thus,

TABLE 5.6 Differences between schizophrenia and personality disorder

	Schizophrenia	Personality disorder
History	Onset in late teens/20s, although 'socially awkward' as a child	'Difficult' traits apparent in childhood or adolescent
	Clear *change* in manner/mental state	Continuous pattern of behaviour/symptoms
Symptoms	Positive, e.g. delusions, hallucinations and/or	Poor impulse control; 'voice-like experiences' rather than true hallucinations
	Negative, e.g. anhedonia	
Behaviour	Usually withdrawn or perplexed	Rule-breaking and self-willed
Mood	Lacking self-confidence and depressive-like	Blames others, labile and/or imposing or demanding
Insight	Often do not see themselves as ill	See themselves as ill rather than behaving inappropriately
Clinician's reaction	Recognizable symptoms, e.g. incoherent or delusional; 'that praecox feeling'	Feel manipulated, irritable and ineffective

with an onset in childhood or adolescence (so history-taking becomes the heart of the matter). The definition also includes notions of a 'deeply ingrained, maladaptive pattern' of character development, from which both individuals and society suffers. Psychotic symptoms, such as hallucinations, do not occur just in the context of personality disorder.

The dilemma is that many patients with very difficult schizophrenic illnesses that seem to have had an early onset (i.e. in their teens) and seem to require regular hospitalization also have personality disorder traits. There is thus a magnifying of the overlap between the two conditions in terms of the experience of the acute mental health ward and the community mental health team. By definition, these teams deal with the more difficult individuals, who will have, alongside their schizophrenic illness, a lack of insight, limited impulse control and/or a tendency to abuse drugs. Because schizophrenia really is an illness, whereas personality disorder is more of a variation on a particular character type, it should not be surprising that the two can overlap.

5.23 What is meant by the term 'borderline personality disorder'?

A number of patients, whether presenting in the GP surgery or at a psychiatric hospital on an acute basis, seem to have psychotic symptoms (e.g. a voice talking to them or paranoid ideation). When the patient is first encountered, part of the differential diagnosis is a schizophrenic illness. Clarifying the history, ideally by getting someone (e.g. a sibling or parent) to give an objective report, may well, however, lead to a diagnosis of a borderline personality disorder. The core features of having a 'borderline' state include impulsive actions, 'outbursts of intense anger' and what is termed 'emotional instability', namely the tendency to over-react, angrily or with tears, to a range of life stressors. More importantly, patients find it hard to know themselves, or may even hate themselves, and have a dread of being abandoned. This internal emptiness leads them to rather intense but not very reliable relationships, ready self-harm (e.g. self-cutting) and a resort to drugs or alcohol in times of crisis. There is no persistent expression of schizophrenic symptoms such as delusions or hallucinations, although when patients are influenced by drugs or alcohol, there may be difficulties in clarifying this.

As with so many other conditions associated with schizophrenia, admission to a properly staffed, well-organized acute inpatient ward, even for a few days, can quickly clarify the borderline diagnosis by observation, proper history-taking and regular mental state assessment. If this cannot be done, diagnostic doubts will persist, to the patient's detriment. Preventing repeated readmission every time a crisis occurs soon becomes the major difficulty, and dealing with it often requires considerable therapeutic skill.

5.24 Are many homicides caused by patients with schizophrenia?

One of the most interesting pieces of research to arise over the past 2 or 3 years has studied the number of homicides associated with schizophrenic patients.[11] The figures remain uncertain in that although patients with schizophrenia do have a slightly higher risk of committing homicide, this depends greatly on the context. In the 1950s, about 40% or more of homicides were committed by so-called 'mentally disordered offenders', that is to say people shown to have a mental disorder (not necessarily schizophrenia) at trial. By the late 1990s, this figure had fallen to below 5%, the actual number being about the same (about 20 a year) but the difference being brought about by the rising tide of 'normal' homicides. In the era of community care, therefore, the chance of being killed by someone who is psychotic compared to someone who is normal but, for example, drunk has been much reduced.

Unfortunately, if someone with schizophrenia commits a murder, the story is often spread all over the front page of the newspapers. This leads to a persisting fear that there is somehow an association between schizophrenia and murder, further stigmatizing many patients and their families. The current anti-stigma campaign ('Every Family in the Land') of the Royal College of Psychiatrists is aimed at dealing with this particular problem. Although not denying that a few patients with schizophrenia do commit murder – usually as a result of strange, threatening symptoms such as the belief that people are interfering with their minds or are out to harm them – it is not uncommon for such patients *also* to have other problems such as a personality disorder, a drink or drug addiction, or an extremely deprived upbringing (*see also refs 12 and 13*).

5.25 Are paedophiles usually schizophrenic?

No. There is no established relationship between patients with schizophrenia and individuals who have a sexual preference for under-age children. Some schizophrenic patients may be vulnerable individuals, easily teased or exploited by delinquent teenagers and thus perceived as potential paedophiles. As a category, however, paedophiles have no obvious psychotic symptoms, merely having a particular sexual preference. Patients with schizophrenia may have clumsy social skills, for example exposing themselves when aroused (and when ill), but have no specific preference for younger people. Unfortunately, if there is a local paedophile witch-hunt, patients with schizophrenia, known to be 'odd' or to have caused problems in the past, may well be targeted.

5.26 Do many drug addicts have schizophrenia?

Although the great majority of those suffering from drug dependence, of whatever form, do not have a schizophrenic illness, the reverse is not true. Thus, in urban areas, 30–50% of schizophrenic patients have a significant alcohol or drug dependence syndrome. This may be because of enhanced anxiety, an attempt to suppress symptoms or even an attempt to 'wash out my brain', as memorably explained by one particular patient using cocaine. Such drug usage can best be seen as a misguided attempt at self-medication and usually involves cannabis, 'crack' or alcohol.

Nevertheless, the great majority of patients with primary drug addiction syndromes, for example to heroin, will not have any significant psychotic symptoms. They may intermittently talk about a 'voice' or 'voices' as part of an attempt to explain their problem or perhaps to gain admission for social relief, but these are only rarely the true hallucinations of a psychosis.

5.27 Can people be paranoid without being schizophrenic?

This is certainly true (*see Q. 1.26*). The term 'paranoid' in itself, as used by the public, generally means a sense of being followed, harassed or looked at in a troubling or even threatening way. Technically, it means more than that, embracing a general sense of making the coincidental seem especially significant. Such paranoia can occur as part of the enhanced self-consciousness of panic attacks, as part of a personality trait, as part of a response to certain drugs (e.g. amphetamines and cannabis) or in association with physical disorders such as hypothyroidism or excessive steroid usage (*Case vignette 5.2*). Loss of social relationships and a personality decline are typical features, as best outlined in the group of 'delusional disorders', described in *Q. 5.13* and *Box 5.1*.

CASE VIGNETTE 5.2

A 38-year-old man was referred after being charged with criminal damage. The incident related to his starting drinking whisky at around 1 p.m. and then, for no reason, walking out into the street with two hammers and smashing up a parked car. The police were called and found him back in his kitchen washing his hands when they arrived. Asked why he had done this, he said he felt he had been in some sense hypnotized and denied any other abnormal experiences. He could give no real reason for his action.

In terms of the man's history, he admitted to having become increasingly fearful about going out in the streets over the past 2 or 3 years. He even, intermittently, carried knives to protect himself. On several occasions, he had become involved in fights, always in the context of heavy alcohol consumption. In terms of his upbringing, he had had problems at school, often truanting, he married young, and he had settled down for some 3 years in a country area of Somerset. The marriage broke up when he was 23, and he then lived rough before moving to London. He obtained various jobs, usually in the catering or bar trade, and admitted to an increasing alcohol intake over the past 5 years.

He described his life overall as 'a jigsaw', with patchy memories of what was going on. An estimated consumption of a bottle of whisky a day was compounded by the intermittent usage of illicit drugs such as amphetamines. He admitted to 'the horrors' (i.e. withdrawal symptoms) on several occasions.

The man's mental state was characterized by his being friendly and cooperative but somewhat anxious and perplexed when trying to clarify his background and experiences. He was reasonably dressed and there was no evidence of depressive symptoms, but he described regular ideas of reference, that is to say the feeling that people were looking at him in the street, and even a sense of number plates having possible significance for him. He denied any hallucinations, such as voices or seeing visions, but described an intermittent sense of being 'hypnotized' or even 'programmed' when drinking. The man agreed that these experiences did not occur when he had not been drinking, and he agreed to attend Alcoholics Anonymous and receive alcohol counselling.

After initially responding to this programme, with no further untoward incidents over the course of the next 6 months, the man moved to another part of the country and was lost to contact. The agreed diagnosis was of an alcohol dependence syndrome in the context of paranoid personality traits.

5.28 Are there any special investigations or tests to separate out the different psychotic illnesses?

In the formal sense of biochemical, radiological or haematological investigations, there are no tests that can separate out any psychotic illness. It is possible for us to exclude organic bases to psychotic symptoms, for example by an EEG (temporal lobe epilepsy), by urinary drug screens or even by assessing autoimmune function in systemic lupus erythematosus. From the other point of view, there are as yet no specific investigations that identify particular illnesses or can separate out manic depression from delusional disorder or schizophrenia. These diagnoses remain essentially clinical, hence the importance of a good mental state examination and regular observations with corroboration of the history. It is extremely likely that reliable tests will appear over the next 10–20 years.

PATIENT QUESTIONS

5.29 How do I know I've really got schizophrenia?

Given the various symptoms that people can have, it is often quite difficult to accept that you really do have a schizophrenic illness. Not only can experiences seem quite real, for example the voices having a very human quality, but it is also frightening to think that you may be 'out of control' or even 'going mad'. There are, however, a number of easily available leaflets or booklets, from the Royal College of Psychiatrists and the organizations MIND and SANE, which provide straightforward accounts of typical symptoms. They will also tell you of the kinds of test that need to be done to exclude any possible physical causes, although these are really uncommon (*see Appendix 2*).

Talking over the issue with someone you trust – your GP, your local nurse or even your local priest – can also be helpful. One should not be afraid to talk about experiences to people (even though this might seem a bit embarrassing) because that is the only way that doctors can be clear about what is the matter and start the right treatment. It is also important to understand that feeling depressed is often caused by some other underlying worry, for example a fear that things are being done to you, and again the right treatment is needed to get rid of that depression.

It must be emphasized that there is no particular blood test or X-ray that can in itself definitively diagnose schizophrenia, although researchers are hunting hard for something reliably diagnostic. Nevertheless, a properly trained doctor can make the diagnosis on the pattern of symptoms and how they affect you just as reliably as when using blood tests for other diseases.

5.30 Should all patients with schizophrenia have some kind of brain scan?

There has been quite a debate about investigations such as CT brain scans, or nowadays MRI scans, in patients with schizophrenia. Given that we consider such illnesses very much to be forms of subtle brain disorder, it seems logical to use these tests. However, no one has yet found any specific abnormality on a CT or MRI scan that can clearly show whether or not you have schizophrenia so there is usually no clinical or treatment benefit in doing one. The scans are also quite costly and can be quite frightening – some people panic in a scanner because of being so closed in, so doing one may be rather distressing.

There are of course a number of research studies underway that are using computerized assessments of large groups of these scans and looking for very subtle differences overall. These may also prove useful at some future date, when reviewed with the benefits of hindsight or to look for any changes over the course of time. Of course, if your doctors are concerned that there may be some other brain abnormality, for example a tumour or a cyst – and other tests or examinations, for example a physical examination, may point to this – it is worth doing such a scan. This is, however, rare, and it is important to emphasize that such scans are not needed to confirm the diagnosis of schizophrenia.

Some researchers have also used what is called 'functional imaging', whereby you are given an injection (or even an inhalation) of radioactive tracer chemicals. Special detectors then pick up the brain's metabolic activity or blood flow (e.g. in positron emission tomography, or PET), and maps or pictures of the brain are made while you (the subject) are carrying out some mental task. These studies are difficult and costly, but we are gradually starting to understand where the brain may be abnormal when a particular symptom (e.g. hallucinations) is occurring.

Management of schizophrenia: drug treatment

6

6.1   Is medication always necessary in the treatment of schizophrenia?

Long-term studies of schizophrenia have shown that only about 10% of those diagnosed as having a schizophrenic illness can remain stable, at least in social and personal terms, without medication. The problem is that this cannot be predicted for any particular type of presentation or pattern of symptoms. The accepted view is therefore that medication remains the cornerstone of successful treatment in schizophrenia, without which other treatments, be they psychological or social, cannot really work. The history of the illness from the pre-pharmacological age is one of crowded asylums, chronic and distressing symptoms, and a form of 'secondary dementia', leading to loss of personal skills, incontinence, mutism and a high level of dependence. Ensuring adherence to medication, and methods of establishing 'compliance', are the essence of best practice.

6.2   Is there any particular medication that stands out from all the others?

No. The recent guidance from the National Institute for Clinical Excellence (NICE) has suggested that 'atypical' antipsychotics are probably the first-line treatment of choice, but no particular drug has been singled out. In addition, there is no evidence that the efficacy of 'atypical' medications is any greater than the traditional dopamine-blocking drugs (such as chlorpromazine) in dealing with symptoms. Whichever one is used, up to 70% of patients will, depending on the length and severity of their illness, respond with a partial or complete remission. Because of their apparently cleaner side-effect profile, the atypical agents are preferred, and it is thought – but not yet proven – that improved compliance should be a particular advantage of the newer drugs.

6.3   Are there any medications without side-effects?

Probably not. As with most drugs in the therapeutic armamentarium, there exists what is known as a therapeutic index. In practical terms, this is the difference in dosage between what will produce a beneficial, therapeutic response and what will generate a 'toxic' effect. This 'toxic' effect may be one or more unpleasant side-effects or may even lead to significant mortality. The dosage range outlined in the *British National Formulary* (*BNF*) is a core guide to safe prescribing, and most antipsychotic drugs are very safe in terms of toxicity if used within these limits. The use of dopamine-blockers can, however, lead to side-effects even at fairly small doses in those sensitive to their impact on muscular or movement control. Virtually all antipsychotic drugs, of whatever class, seem to confer a degree of sedation, of a subtle or obvious type, and weight gain is not uncommon. It is generally accepted that having an honest but not alarmist discussion about these possible problems is an essential part of the preparation for treatment.

6.4 What's the best drug to start treating someone with schizophrenia?

There is no 'best' medication, given that all medications have equal efficacy. However, availability, the patient's attitude to medication and aspects of the presentation – are they withdrawn or are they agitated? – will influence the clinician's choice. The commonly prescribed medications in two main classes of antipsychotic drug – atypical and typical – are outlined in *Table 6.1*. This assumes that the patient is willing to take medication orally and prefers so to do. Many of the drugs are available not only as tablets, but also as syrups or easily soluble preparations, and developing clinical experience with one or two of either class is the best practice. Supplementing with benzodiazepines, or providing additional medication – on a 'as required' (p.r.n.) basis to deal with side-effects – is also part and parcel of good management Trying to stick to a single medication is of course always worthwhile but may not be possible in agitated states. Assuming a definite diagnosis, such treatment can readily be started in primary care. Obtaining an additional specialist opinion is probably a must in order to reassure the family and obtain specialist support in ongoing management.

6.5 What is the best treatment for acute schizophrenia if the patient is very agitated?

This will depend on whether the patient is compliant with medication – i.e. willing to take an oral preparation – or refuses so to do. All antipsychotics are calming, hence their formal description as 'major tranquillizers', but chlorpromazine is particularly so because of its wide range of activity (i.e. it is also antihistaminic and anti-adrenergic). The dose (50–100 mg 3–4 times a day) can be fine-tuned every 2 or 3 hours, and because of its in-built anticholinergic effect it is less likely to generate side-effects in the short term. Supplementing with benzodiazepines (diazepam 5–10 mg or lorazepam 2 mg) reduces arousal, helps with sleep and is again very flexible in its dosage. The use of immediate, relatively high doses of atypical agents, along with benzodiazepines, is now also being recommended (especially to

TABLE 6.1 Commonly prescribed oral medications for the treatment of schizophrenia (proprietary names)

Typical (dopamine blockade)			Atypical (5-hydroxytryptamine effect +/– limited dopamine blockade)		
	Usual daily dose	Maximum dose		Usual daily dose	Maximum dose
Chlorpromazine	100–800 mg	1 g	Olanzapine	5–20 mg	20–25 mg
Haloperidol	5–30 mg	60–80 mg	Quetiapine°	100–500 mg	750 mg
Trifluoperazine	5–30 mg	30 mg	Amisulpride	40–800 mg	1.2 g
Pimozide*	2–20 mg	20 mg	Risperidone†	2–6 mg	16 mg
Sulpiride	200–1600 mg	2.4 g	Clozapine°	200–400 mg	900 mg
Zuclopenthixol	20–50 mg	150 mg	Zotepine	100–200 mg	300 mg

*ECG required before treatment; †has dopamine blockade side-effects above this dosage; °requires regular haematological monitoring

avoid side-effects), but more evidence on the efficacy of this approach is required, and the flexibility of 3–4 times a day dosage may not be available.

If injectable preparations are required for a resistant patient, transfer to hospital (under the Mental Health Act if necessary) is vital. Lorazepam 2–4 mg given intramuscularly is safe, effective in sedation and short-acting, while haloperidol 5–10 mg intramuscularly can also be used, either to supplement the lorazepam or on its own. A close monitoring of such patients' physical and mental state is a priority, as is the early use of intramuscular (or oral) anticholinergics such as procyclidine 5–10 mg to counteract any side-effects (e.g. acute dystonia).

6.6 If starting treatment with a typical medication, how readily can one switch to an atypical agent if there are side-effects?

As many doctors are rather more familiar, particularly at the primary care level, with traditional medications such as chlorpromazine and haloperidol, many patients, particularly if they are agitated, will have been started on these. This is perfectly good practice provided the side-effects are monitored closely. Initiating treatment with atypical agents in quieter, more compliant patients is – based on our current knowledge – worth encouraging, but these drugs are not entirely free of side-effects, and some patients simply do not respond to one class or the other.

When switching from a typical drug – Box 6.1 outlining reasons for and against switching medication – such as chlorpromazine to an atypical agent, there is no need for a 'washout' period. It is usually best to build up the atypical agent to full dosage over the course of several weeks while continuing with, for example, the chlorpromazine and then gradually withdrawing the latter. Likewise, with a switch from an atypical to a typical

---

BOX 6.1 Switching medications in schizophrenia

Reasons for:

Intolerable side-effects

Partial or full resistance to
treatment

Relapse or worsening of symptoms

Patient/family request

Physical/psychiatric complications

Known to be non-compliant

Reasons against:

Poor insight or no clear reason

Successful treatment

When dosage adjustment may
suffice

Major life changes are ongoing

Drug/alcohol abuse or risk of
violence

---

drug, building up the latter to a regular dosage over the course of a week or
two and then gradually withdrawing the atypical agent is the safest practice.
The main problem will be sedation, and both patient and family will need
to have this temporary problem fully explained to them (*see refs 13 and 14*).

6.7   What are the common side-effects of 'typical' antipsychotic drugs?

 These are outlined in *Box 6.2*, most being the consequences of dopamine
blockade. The three major areas of side-effects are therefore associated with
lack of drive/sedation, sexual difficulties (as a result of a raised prolactin
level with the release from inhibitory dopamine control) and movement
disorders. Depending on the dosages used, such effects will occur in
30–70% of patients, some being more obvious than others. Abnormal
movements can be monitored clinically and scored on standard rating
scales (e.g. Abnormal Involuntary Movements Scale), whereas others, for
example, erectile problems may need sensitive questioning to elicit them.
There are also drug-specific problems (e.g. a sun-induced rash with
chlorpromazine) and a host of minor idiosyncratic reactions (see the most
recent *BNF*).

6.8   What's the best way of treating these side-effects?

 Assuming one cannot lower the dosage or change medication, which are the
best practical approaches if possible, the treatment of side-effects will
generally require anticholinergic medications (for movement disorders) or
sometimes beta-blockers (e.g. propranolol) or benzodiazepines. Acute
dystonia (use intravenous or intramuscular procyclidine if severe) and
parkinsonism usually respond well to anticholinergic drugs (e.g.
Procyclidine 5–10 mg up to three times daily, or orphenadrine 50–100 mg
up to three times a day); akathisia is often less responsive. Propranolol
(40–80 mg up to three times daily) and/or benzodiazepines (e.g. diazepam
50–10 mg up to three times a day) may be more effective in this regard. The

> **BOX 6.2 Side-effects of dopamine-blocking drugs (class specific)**
>
> **Sedation**
>
> Loss of drive and 'get up and go'
> Drowsiness and hypersomnia
> Loss of concentration and initiative
> Feeling 'drugged' and 'flat'
>
> *Sexual*
>
> Loss of libido
> Erectile failure (partial or full)
> Delayed or absent ejaculation
> Anorgasmia (in women)
> Inappropriate lactation
>
> *Movement*
>
> Acute dystonia (especially face or jaw)
> Akathisia (inability to sit still)
> Parkinsonism (tremor, bradykinesia, cogwheel rigidity)
> Tardive dyskinesia (late onset, variable range of movements)

later-onset condition known as tardive dyskinesia is usually resistant to such approaches, although an increased dosage of the dopamine blocker may abolish it (probably, however, to the detriment of the patient's mental state because of sedation).

Alternatively, giving lower doses of medication while supplementing with benzodiazepines can maintain stability in terms of the mental state yet make patients feel physically more comfortable. Switching completely to atypical antipsychotic medications, if that is an option and they have not previously been shown to be ineffective, is nowadays an obvious alternative measure. These of course have their own side-effects (*see Q. 3.10*), which need to be acknowledged.

6.9 Can benzodiazepines or other tranquillizers be helpful in the treatment of schizophrenia?

Yes, they are very helpful. Not only are benzodiazepines such as lorazepam and diazepam useful in early, agitated states, particularly if patients require sedation on inpatient units, but they can also be of continuing use for those with an added anxiety component, this being a problem for up to a third of patients. Benzodiazepines can help lower arousal, thus reducing the requirement for higher doses of antipsychotics, they can promote sleep, and they can help with some movement disorders, such as akathisia or tremor. Concerns about dependence need to be viewed within the context of patients who are going to be taking major tranquillizers for a long time. Continuing or intermittent benzodiazepine usage is highly unlikely to generate dependence behaviours. Standard preparations such as diazepam, with its wide dosage range, and nitrazepam, with its long half-life (especially helpful for sleeping), are the most practical in this respect.

6.10 What are the usual side-effects of atypical medications?

Despite being clean in terms of movement disorder – although these have occasionally been reported – atypical agents tend to be sedating in some individuals, sometimes producing a rather marked degree of somnolence. Most of them are also associated with a tendency, in a third or more of patients, to put on weight, which can sometimes be quite distressing, although it does level off. Concerns have also been raised about the development of hyperglycaemia or frank type 2 (non-insulin-dependent) diabetes, ECG abnormalities and (specifically with clozapine) forms of anaemia. The details of side-effects are listed in *Box 6.3*.

6.11 Are any particular drugs effective for any particular symptoms?

There is no evidence that any specific antipsychotic drug is especially effective for hallucinations, for example, or thought broadcast or other forms of thought interference. If a drug is effective, it will generally be effective across the spectrum of 'positive' symptoms, and there is no evidence that using additional drugs will enhance the response. It should also be emphasized that both 'typical' and 'atypical' types of antipsychotic are really effective only for positive symptoms, and the evidence for their reducing 'negative' symptoms is very limited. There may be an apparent improvement using atypical agents because over-sedation or parkinsonian effects (e.g. a somewhat unchanging facial expression) are no longer present. Better compliance may likewise reduce certain symptoms, for example thought broadcast (feeling that people can read your mind), as these are likely to enhance the social withdrawal and limited speech so typical of the negative symptom group.

BOX 6.3	Side-effects of atypical medication
Sedation	Daytime drowsiness, hypersomnia, loss of drive, impaired concentration, postural hypotension
Metabolic	Weight gain, enhanced appetite +/- craving for carbohydrates, hyperglycaemia (especially clozapine)

In a more general sense, patients who are aroused and anxious often benefit from drugs such as chlorpromazine that have additional anxiolytic properties, whereas those who are withdrawn or rather sluggish will do better on a drug such as trifluoperazine (from the typical group). Such differential secondary effects are not especially apparent for the atypical drugs, although clozapine and olanzapine seem to be often slightly more sedating (and therefore anxiety-relieving?) than the others. The rule is, however, to take account of individual variation in response and thus tailor the medication to an individual's own pattern of symptoms and side-effects.

6.12 Can the newer medications ('atypicals') help with negative symptoms?

There continues to be a debate over this, part of which will depend on how the negative symptoms are characterized. Some studies show a limited improvement in negative symptom score on standard scales such as the Positive and Negative Symptoms Scale, but these differences are often not very large. They may reflect better compliance, and thus an improvement in underlying 'positive' symptoms such as intrusive voices, or they may reflect reduced sedation. There is a little evidence to support a modern version of sulpiride (called amisulpride), but corroborating research is still required. The strongest evidence base relates to the use of clozapine in patients with chronic resistant schizophrenia, which usually includes a degree of negative symptomatology, but this again usually works by reducing the intensity of positive symptoms. The use of antidepressants on a trial basis, given the big overlap in clinical assessment between 'depressive' and 'negative' symptoms, is well worth considering.

6.13 Are patients more compliant with any particular medications or forms of treatment?

Compliance with medication, now often termed 'adherence', is a major problem throughout medicine but particularly in the treatment of psychotic illnesses. Depending on a patient's upbringing, intelligence and insight into their illness, certain treatments may make more sense than others. Some patients prefer syrups to tablets; others prefer tablets to injections or vice versa. If a medication helps with a particular symptom, for example difficulty sleeping, patients will happily take it. If it also, for example, relieves headaches or reduces anxiety (secondary to paranoid beliefs), that is likewise a positive reinforcer.

Unpleasant effects, for example muscle spasms or not being able to attain an erection, will quite quickly put patients off. Remember too that whereas a third of 'refusers' cite side-effects as the reason for their refusal, doctors tend to recognize fewer than 10% of such concerns! The use of formal 'compliance training' tries to clarify these matters, and warning patients of temporary side-effects, explaining the rationale of medication and trying to fit medication to an individual's needs are all part of good practice.

Simply listing the good and bad aspects of taking a particular drug can start this dialogue off. The benefit of the greater range of antipsychotics now available, particularly with the atypical agents, is that a drug suited to an individual's reactions is more readily found. We still await formal studies showing that there is better compliance with atypical medications, although this is the general clinical impression.

6.14 Why do so many patients stop taking their medications?

Medication can be stopped because of side-effects, lack of insight, sheer forgetfulness, outside influences or simply patients feeling so well that they think they are 'cured'. The most distressing side-effects include excessive sedation, muscle spasms and tremors, weight gain and sexual difficulties. Insight is a particular problem for those who do not believe they are or have been ill (which affects at least 50% of patients), whereas all of us tend to forget to take our medications, particularly if the regime is a bit complicated or the drugs are to be taken more than once a day. There are also, unfortunately, many individuals or groups who do not 'believe' in medication, considering it to be addictive, unnecessary, less valuable than 'counselling' or less efficacious than the right diet, religious invocations or other alternative treatments. Finally, some individuals just feel so well that they do not believe they need to continue with medication, a belief reinforced by standard health advice (e.g. taking antibiotics for only a week or 10 days) and the difficulty of distinguishing a 'cure' from maintenance therapy.

6.15 Are there any particular ways of improving compliance?

Getting patients to take medication is half the trick of psychiatric practice. The following rules generally apply (*see also Box 7.4*).

- Explain the nature of the illness to the patient and family without using euphemisms. Do, however, use the information packs or leaflets provided by voluntary organizations and the Royal College of Psychiatrists.
- Try to explain the role of medication. Emphasize that the illness is a physical problem of 'the nerves' or even 'brain chemicals' rather than a moral defect or something to be ashamed of.

■ Warn about and monitor side-effects closely, adapting dosages and/or medications to make the patient as comfortable as possible.

■ Use simple, once- or twice-daily regimes if possible rather than complicated prescribing approaches.

■ Involve the family and/or carers in this approach and provide support for them as well if necessary.

■ A formal, cognitive-behavioural approach to insight can show significant improvements, using trained nurses able to deliver a psycho-educational programme to both patient and family. The best programmes seem to cut the relapse rate by 20–30%.

■ If necessary, engage an Assertive Outreach Team (as promoted by the NHS Plan and National Service Framework), and be prepared to use the Mental Health Act to insist on continued treatment since patients do have a 'right' to care.

6.16 What are the indications for starting people on depot injections?

Persistent relapse on oral medication, because of forgetfulness or non-compliance, or a need to maintain medication (e.g. because of at-risk behaviours when patients become unwell) are the usual indicators for using depot injections. A number of patients prefer them since there is much less hassle involved in having an injection every 3–4 weeks than in taking tablets two or three times a day. Furthermore, lower dosage can in general be used since injections avoid the 'first-pass metabolism' of the liver (which removes over 90% of the active agent!), the drug going essentially straight into the blood stream. Patients under longer-term Mental Health Act orders (such as a restriction order under Section 41) are particularly well managed by depot injections because of the certainty of dose and prescribing, and (coincidentally?) because of the regular contact with the patient by a trained nurse (*see Table 6.2*). Again, there is no reason why GPs should not initiate depot treatment while engaging the specialist team to help to monitor effects and side-effects.

6.17 Are expensive newer drugs really worth prescribing?

There has been considerable debate around this issue over the past few years, but the cost-effectiveness data are increasingly showing that it is cheaper to keep people out of hospital than to give them the wrong medication. The mental health budget is dominated by inpatient care, which absorbs some 70–80% of all costs. A medication that a patient will accept, that does not have side-effects and that is easy to administer is well worth it in terms of avoiding such expenses. Furthermore, while these drugs may be expensive now, they will soon be out of patent, and the relative cost

TABLE 6.2 Depot preparations for schizophrenia (intramuscular)

Equivalents (BNF)	Trade name	Proprietary name	Recommended dosage	Test dose
200	Clopixol	Zuclopenthixol decanoate	200–600 mg every 1–4 weeks	100 mg
40	Depixol	Flupenthixol decanoate	50–400 mg every 1–4 weeks	20 mg
100	Haldol	Haloperidol decanoate	50–300 mg every 2–4 weeks	25–50 mg
25	Modecate	Fluphenazine decanoate	25–150 mg every 2–4 weeks	12.5 mg
50	Piportil	Pipothiazine palmitate	50–200 mg every 2–4 weeks	25 mg

N.B. All of these preparations are given via deep intramuscular injection, ideally into the gluteal musculature by a trained nurse

Short-acting depot preparation
Clopixol Acuphase (zuclopenthixol acetate) 50–150 mg every 3 days (maximum dosage 400 mg via a maximum of four injections)

of all psychiatric medications, compared with some modern antibiotics, angiotensin-converting enzyme inhibitors or HIV treatments, is actually very small. In the broader conspectus of prescribing costs, antipsychotic medications, apart from clozapine (approximately £2000–4000 per annum, largely because of the safety requirements and blood testing) are really not a major factor.

6.18 How long does medication take to become effective?

In terms of a genuine antipsychotic effect, whether with a typical or an atypical agent, antipsychotics usually take up to a month to eliminate (or start to eliminate) active, positive symptoms. Some patients will of course start to feel better within a few days, particularly if they feel calmer and less anxious because of the sedating effect. Other individuals may take up to 3 months or even more to improve, and the current NICE recommendation to change medications (if ineffective) after a couple of months is probably unrealistic for those people who have been ill for a long time. In essence, the longer the illness, the longer it will take to get people better, so someone who has been unwell for 2 or 3 years, slowly deteriorating in the community, is unlikely to get fully better within 1 or 2 months.

6.19 If a medication isn't effective, what should one do next?

There are a number of standard algorithms outlined by various research groups detailing what to do if medications are not effective. Assuming that one has started with an atypical agent and used it at a full dosage for at least 1 or 2 months, without even a partial alleviation of symptoms, it is worth considering an alternative. Patients clearly need close monitoring, either via standard rating scales (e.g. the Brief Psychiatric Rating Scale) or via careful clinical assessment. Compliance should always be carefully reviewed.

The next step is to switch to a typical antipsychotic, again at the fullest dosage possible, monitoring its effects. If side-effects are the limiting factor, alternatives of either can be used to circumvent the problem. If one has used at least two drugs, either alone or in combination, or more usually three or four of the standard medications, without any significant improvement (i.e. there is resistant schizophrenia), clozapine is the drug of choice. Every unit should have a standard algorithm looking at alternatives before reaching clozapine, but such treatment should not be delayed for too long because the longer the active illness, the more uncertain the prognosis. Three standard algorithms are outlined in *Figures 6.1–6.3* for maintenance, poor response and treatment-intolerant patients.

6.20 Is it reasonable to combine typical and atypical medications?

All the official handouts say that one should not do this, but in fact, in the 'dirty' clinical situation, this can sometimes be helpful. For example, a patient who has side-effects when taking depot medication can be put on a lower dosage, with a supplementary atypical agent, thus maximizing their response and minimizing side-effects. Furthermore, if non-compliance or semi-compliance is a problem, the regular depot administration provides a safety measure, particularly if relapse means at-risk behaviours such as self-neglect or violence. Alternatively, the use of drugs such as chlorpromazine simply to help with sleep, alongside, perhaps, a standard atypical drug, can help with a specific symptom or problem, again enhancing quality of life and compliance. It is clearly best practice to try to avoid combinations and multiple prescribing, but in the end the particular patient's needs should remain paramount.

6.21 What if the patient does not get better despite trying two or three different medications?

As outlined in *Q. 6.19*, every psychiatric unit should have guidelines on how to progress in terms of providing treatment. It is most important to review compliance (blood levels being available for some drugs), if necessary using

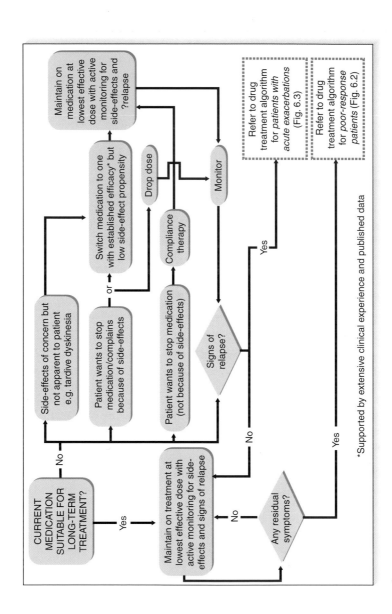

Fig. 6.1 Drug treatment algorithm for patients on maintenance therapy.

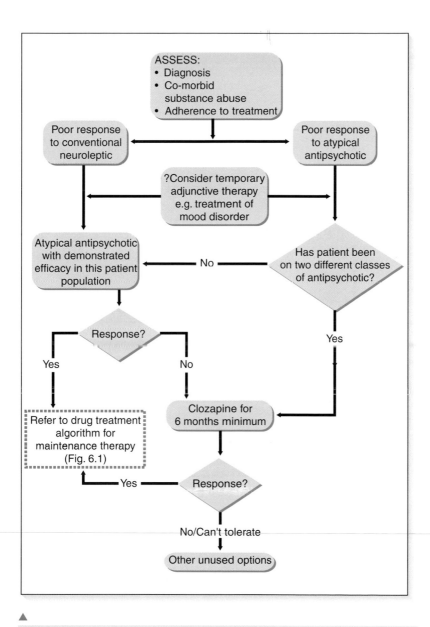

Fig. 6.2 Drug treatment algorithm for poor-reponse patients.

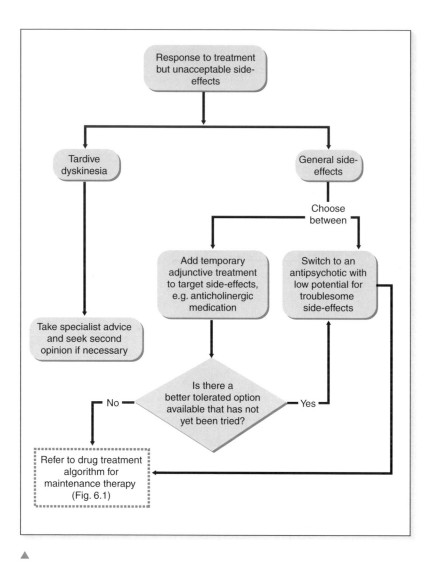

Fig. 6.3 Drug treatment algorithm for treatment-intolerant patients.

an inpatient admission to check this (as well as to check the diagnosis as organic problems and personality disorders can fool even the best clinicians). The use of depot preparations rather than oral medication can (sometimes surprisingly) be extremely helpful in some patients, and a urinary drug screen (is the patient taking amphetamines or cocaine, on a regular basis, for example?) can also clarify some clinical situations. True resistant schizophrenia means that one has to consider clozapine, and a specialist clozapine clinic (*Box 6.4*) is usually a desirable resource given its complexities (weekly blood testing at first, closely monitored prescribing, and screening for other side-effects; *Case vignette 6.1*). Clozapine cannot currently be prescribed in general practice.

CASE VIGNETTE 6.1

A 38-year-old Chinese woman who had come to England 5 years previously was brought to the psychiatric emergency clinic by her family. She had in fact been 'ill' before emigrating and had received a combination of traditional medications (chlorpromazine) and herbal remedies while in the Far East. A key symptom was of regular voices, constantly talking about her and to her, and plaguing her with their presence. She attributed these to long-dead ancestors, sent to haunt her for her sins, and made several serious suicide attempts, including jumping out of a second-floor window. She had to be admitted under Section 3 of the Mental

---

BOX 6.4 A specialist clozapine clinic

- Clozapine can be prescribed only by specialist clinicians registered with the Clozaril Patient Monitoring Service
- Regular blood tests (full blood count) must be coordinated with pharmacy prescribing
- Unless a 'green' blood count is received, the pharmacy cannot prescribe
- Blood tests are required weekly (for 18 weeks), then fortnightly (for 1 year) and then monthly (ad infinitum)
- Patients need to attend for blood tests (+/– clozapine level), provision of medication and regular review (mental state and side-effects)
- A specialist nurse attached to the clinic can supervise, monitor and help with advice on all aspects of care
- There are many common but transient side-effects, e.g. tremor, dizziness, headache, hyper/hypotension (on drug initiation), sedation, nausea and seizures (with higher doses)
- Common persistent side-effects, e.g. weight gain, hypersalivation, constipation and tachycardia, occur, requiring specialist management

Health Act on three different occasions, partially responded to depot medication but was largely unable to care for her children even when she returned home in a relatively stable state. Her husband was initially supportive but became increasingly frustrated by her limited abilities in terms of childcare, her obvious tremor and parkinsonian appearance, and her limited self-care.

After the woman's third admission, it was agreed that, given the length of her illness and the chronicity of her symptoms – she continued to hear voices even when on medication – she should be offered clozapine. Her limited English required a Chinese support worker to help in explaining the protocols (e.g. regular blood tests) to her and to ensure that she took medication on a regular basis. Initiation of the drug began in hospital, and over the course of a 3-month admission, she gradually improved to a significant degree. She described her head becoming clearer and the voices fading, and even her appearance changed. She was much smarter in her grooming and self-care, was able to communicate better with her family and children, and lost her secondary depressive symptoms. Some 2 years after starting clozapine, she was back living with her family, no longer troubled by intrusive symptoms and helping to look after her children.

6.22 Are there any other drugs apart from the typical and atypical antipsychotics that can be useful in schizophrenia?

Some patients benefit from antidepressants, and distinguishing between depressive symptoms and negative symptoms is often difficult; a trial of antidepressants may even be worthwhile. Likewise, difficulties in sleeping can be addressed by standard hypnotics, and fears of the regular usage of, for example, benzodiazepines (i.e. minor tranquillizers) should be tempered by the fact that patients are already taking major tranquillizers. Such drugs can help to lower arousal and reduce the need for using higher doses of antipsychotics. The use of mood stabilizers (e.g. lithium, carbamazepine and sodium valproate) is controversial, but if there is clear evidence of mood swings, a trial of a mood stabilizer is again worth considering. Such decisions are best taken by specialist psychiatrists, in terms of examining the mental state and clarifying the diagnosis and symptomatology.

6.23 Is there a role for lithium in the treatment of schizophrenia?

No. A number of clinicians have tried using lithium, alongside antipsychotics, because of a pattern of what looks like mood swings, or even intermittent 'manic' type behaviours, and the differential diagnosis between a lithium-responsive condition such as manic depressive disorder and certain forms of schizophrenia can be quite difficult. There was a vogue for changing diagnoses in the 1960s and 70s simply because lithium was available, but this made clinicians more careful in their diagnostic practice. Given the need for regular blood tests, potential side-effects and established lack of efficacy, the use of lithium in patients who simply have schizophrenia is unjustified.

6.24 Is there a role for anticonvulsants, such as carbamazepine or sodium valproate, in the treatment of schizophrenia?

As with lithium, these drugs are not indicated unless there is a clear indication of mood swings (or even fits, such as from temporal lobe epilepsy). They do have a considerable role in the management of mood swing disorders and have also been used as a generalized form of 'anti-aggression' medication, but reports are again anecdotal, and there is no current justification for their use in straightforward schizophrenia.

6.25 Is there any justification for going beyond the BNF dosage limits?

Going beyond the *BNF* is sometimes justifiable provided one is quite clear about the diagnosis, has monitored the effects of all dosages, has confirmed compliance and is sure there is a reasonable likelihood of an improved effect. Individuals metabolize drugs with remarkable variety, some patients, for example, showing no evidence of an active level of flupenthixol (Depixol; usually given as a depot injection) even on weekly doses. High-dose medication has its risks, particularly in the aroused patient, and one should have a very low threshold for reviewing cardiac status, carrying out an ECG and closely monitoring both the physical and the mental state. Patients not responding to regular doses who do not seem to show any significant side-effects can be cautiously put on higher doses, at least on a trial basis. If improvement occurs, a gradual reduction to a more normal level can often be achieved, maintenance seeming to require less 'heroic' dosing than getting a patient into remission.

6.26 Are there any routine assessments that should be carried out before using antipsychotics?

Given that one is clear about the diagnosis and has eliminated possible alternatives caused by, for example, metabolic conditions (e.g. hypothyroidism, drug abuse and temporal lobe epilepsy), the only assessment that is nowadays probably a 'must' is an ECG. It is, however, good practice to carry out baseline investigations, especially for blood sugar, given the higher rate of diabetes in all patients with schizophrenia and the potential of some of the 'atypical' medications (e.g. clozapine) to enhance that. Using a test dose (e.g. half-strength depot administration) or an initially very low dose for 2 or 3 days of standard neuroleptics is also good practice. Checking the background history in case there is any pre-existing unusual, allergic or other reaction to antipsychotic agents is useful in choosing which particular drug to use. See *Table 6.3* for routine monitoring for clozapine and atypical agents.

TABLE 6.3 Management of treatment-resistant schizophrenia

Drug	Obligatory monitoring		Suggested additional monitoring		Actions
	Baseline	Continuation	Baseline	Continuation	
Clozapine	Full blood count (prescriber and pharmacist must register)	Full blood count weekly for 18 weeks, then at least fortnightly for the first year and monthly thereafter	ECG EEG Liver function tests Urea and electrolytes Blood pressure Creatine phosphokinase Temperature Weight Blood sugar	ECG – when maintenance dose is reached EEG – as above and if myoclonus or seizures occur Liver function tests/urea and electrolytes – every 3–6 months Blood pressure – 4-hourly during initiation Creatine phosphokinase – if neuroleptic malignant syndrome suspected Temperature – daily for the first 3 weeks and then weekly Weight – as needed	Stop clozapine if the neutrophil count is below 1.5×10^9/l Refer to specialist care if the neutrophil count is below 0.5×10^9/l Stop clozapine if the ECG changes or there are signs of heart failure Use sodium valproate if the EEG shows clear epileptiform changes or if seizures occur Stop clozapine if liver function tests indicate hepatitis Monitor closely if the temperature rises
Risperidone	None	None	Blood sugar Full blood count Liver function tests	Full blood count – 3–6 monthly	Stop if neutrophil count is below 1.5×10^9/l
Olanzapine	None	None	Urea and electrolytes Blood pressure	Liver function tests – 3–6 monthly	Use with caution in hepatic or renal failure
Quetiapine	None	None	Prolactin Creatine phosphokinase	Urea and electrolytes 3–6 monthly	Stop if prolactin-related effects are intolerable

TABLE 6.3 Management of treatment-resistant schizophrenia—cont'd

Drug	Obligatory monitoring		Suggested additional monitoring		Actions
	Baseline	Continuation	Baseline	Continuation	
Amisulpride	None	None	Blood sugar level Weight	Blood pressure – frequently during initiation Prolactin – if adverse effects occur Creatine phosphokinase – if neuroleptic malignant syndrome suspected Blood sugar level Weight – as needed	Stop if NMS is suspected

TABLE 6.4 Routine monitoring for patients on atypical antipsychotics: antipsychotic interactions (see *BNF* for details)

	Effect
Alcohol	Enhanced sedative effect
Antacids	Reduced absorption, especially phenothiazines
Analgesics	Enhanced sedation/hypotension (e.g. indomethacin and haloperidol)
Anti-arrhythmics	Risk of arrhythmia, especially pimozide
Antibacterials	Risk of arrhythmia, especially pimozide
Antidepressants	As above and increased antipsychotic plasma concentrations
Anti-epileptics	Accelerated metabolism of the antipsychotic and reduced plasma concentrations
Antihypertensives	Enhanced hypotensive effect
Antivirals	May enhance the plasma concentration of specific antipsychotics
Lithium	Increased risk of extrapyramidal effects

6.27 What important interactions are there with the standard (typical and atypical) antipsychotics?

These drugs are, by and large, very clean and can be used alongside most other medications, whether those used in psychiatric practice or in general medicine. A list of possible interactions is outlined in *Table 6.4*, but it should be emphasized that these are unusual and rather idiosyncratic, and there are no absolute contraindications.

6.28 Can you measure drug levels in the blood routinely?

No. Certain specialist units can do blood level measurements, but variations in individual plasma levels are enormous given the range of different metabolites produced by most antipsychotics. There is no evidence that a particular level in a particular patient is effective or not effective, the most useful assessment being by clinical examination and a review of side-effects. If using typical, dopamine-blocking drugs, a prolactin level, at baseline (pre-medication) and after regular treatment, can indicate the level of dopamine blockade. This is to some extent also a measure of compliance, although not used routinely as such.

The one exception to this rule is the measurement of clozapine levels, which is now quite routine. This both enables compliance to be checked (important in such a difficult drug to use clinically) and ensures the correct dosage as a level of less than 35 ng/ml is usually ineffective. The ability to measure drug levels more closely would certainly enhance the quality of care that could be offered to patients with schizophrenia and should be a priority for the future.

6.29 Is there a role for antidepressants in treating schizophrenia?

Depending on different studies, between 20% and 50% of patients with schizophrenia seem to have something approaching a depressive condition. This may be a combination of genuine depressive symptoms with negative symptoms, or the latter simply mimicking depression. It is also well known that many patients with schizophrenia have been treated for 'depression' before the basis for their depression (i.e. their psychotic symptoms) has been clarified. Nevertheless, regular monitoring of potential depressive symptoms is part of good practice, and a trial of treatment with a standard antidepressant can be worthwhile in patients about whom one is uncertain. No particular group of antidepressants (e.g. tricyclics or selective serotonin reuptake inhibitors) is specifically indicated, but non-sedating medications are probably most useful in patients presenting with lack of drive, lack of motivation and a general slowing down.

6.30 How long should you go on with antipsychotic treatment?

The modern view is that, given the current role and effectiveness of the medications available, treatment is for life. That is not to say that a closely monitored trial of withdrawal should not be undertaken every now and then, with the patient's and family's agreement. In essence, however, antipsychotic treatment is like insulin therapy for diabetes, or thyroxine for hypothyroidism: one needs it as if it were a special 'vitamin' to supplement abnormal neurochemistry. Many clinicians will not use the 'for life' phrase, preferring to suggest that taking medication for up to 5 years at least should be the first aim. Given the possibilities of new treatments being marketed, this seems reasonably honest in terms of clarifying the nature of the condition and helping to enhance compliance.

6.31 Can patients get withdrawal effects from medication?

There are no specific withdrawal effects from antipsychotic agents, apart from a relapse of the symptoms of the illness. If anything, patients feel a little bit 'better' when off medication, particularly if they have been taking traditional antipsychotics, which tend to make them feel a degree of 'psychological parkinsonism' (e.g. lacking drive and sexual interest). This paradoxical 'feeling well window' is often the basis for patients and/or families blaming the illness on the medication. Furthermore, when relapse does occur, as it almost always does, there may have been a gap of 3 or 4 months, or even longer, so the patient does not link discontinuation of medication with getting ill. Other intervening factors, for example a row with a girlfriend or a change of housing, will (not unnaturally) be seen as much more significant.

6.32 What are the best arrangements for managing treatment between GPs and specialist teams (shared care)?

There is always a dilemma over who should prescribe, how patients should be followed up and how GPs communicate with community mental health teams (CMHTs) and consultant psychiatrists. Individual and local preferences will vary, but liaison attachments seem to be the most widely used. These involve a group of GPs meeting the relevant consultants, usually with another specified CMHT member (who acts as a regular liaison between that practice and the CMHT), and discussing clinical management. Problems usually arise when there is a gap in service, that is to say each side thinks the other is, for example, prescribing or monitoring. The Care Programme Approach (CPA) review will usually identify a care coordinator, whose task is to check up on just these concerns. The motto should nevertheless be 'If in doubt, communicate.' Key aspects of such arrangements are summarised in *Box 6.5*.

BOX 6.5 Arrangements for shared care between GPs and the community mental health team (CMHT)

■ Establishment of local agreements on the criteria for referral to, and discharge from, the local CMHT

■ Establish in each practice a case register of those in shared care

■ Clarify who does what – in terms of medication prescribing, medication monitoring, mental state assessment, physical assessment and (if required) blood level monitoring or urinary drug screening

■ Planned and regular communication, via regular liaison meetings, for example reviewing those on the case register

■ Agreeing on a liaison worker from the CMHT for each GP practice (or group of practices if single-handed, for example), with a defined role and tasks

■ Agree on a crisis plan, with relapse indicators if useful and, if practicable, involving advanced directives

■ Agree on the Care Programme Approach (CPA) arrangements, on a regular updating of changes in prescribing, and consider regular audits of care arrangements

PQ   PATIENT QUESTIONS

6.33   Can some patients stop medication without any relapse?

This is a perennial question, asked by many patients and families. Long-term studies show that perhaps 10% of patients seem to stay well – or at least socially stable – without medication, but no one can tell who this will be or what particular symptoms predict such stability. Sadly, most patients relapse on stopping medication, which is actually the commonest cause of relapse and the commonest cause of readmission to hospital. If planning to try to discontinue medication, for whatever reason, it is always best to do it slowly, to let your GP or community psychiatric nurse know and to try to do it while being closely supported. In that way, symptoms can be picked up quickly, medication can be restarted before things get out of hand, and harm can be minimized. It is also worth remembering that every time you become ill, the chances of a full recovery are slightly reduced, each relapse leaving patients with a bit of a 'defect' or even some stronger residual symptom, for example persistent hallucinations. Community care has essentially been made possible by the availability of medication, before which the great majority of patients with schizophrenia spent their lives in hospital.

6.34   What if I fall pregnant when taking medication?

Doctors agree that it is best not to take any medication during pregnancy, especially during the first 3 months (the first 'trimester'), when a growing baby is most at risk. There is, however, absolutely no evidence that traditional antipsychotic drugs cause any harm and, as they have been in use for about 50 years, this evidence is very reliable. Staying on medication, and thereby keeping well during pregnancy, is the best advice, although stopping medication (which should be oral at this stage) for 2–3 days before delivery will reduce the chances of having a rather sedated baby at birth. The same applies to newer 'atypical' drugs, but we have less long-term experience of their effects on babies so switching to a traditional drug might be theoretically safer.

After the birth, it is wisest to go back on your regular treatment – whatever medication you were on – because there is a very high risk of relapse at this time (a form of so-called 'puerperal psychosis'). Since all antipsychotics are found in breast milk, albeit in small amounts, it is probably best not to breastfeed. A full discussion of all these factors with your psychiatrist during pregnancy, to get everything clear in your mind, is the best approach.

6.35   What if I'm being given a very high dose of medication?

This may be because you are not getting better on regular doses or even because you are 'resistant' to medication. The advice of the Royal College of Psychiatrists on doses above the *BNF* upper limit is as follows:

1. Alternative medications and even clozapine may need to be considered.
2. Overweight and elderly patients are especially at risk of side-effects.

3. Regular ECGs should be carried out, and the dose reduced if certain abnormalities are detected.
4. Regular pulse, blood pressure and temperature checks should be performed; those taking the medications should maintain an adequate fluid intake.
5. Doses should be increased only slowly (about weekly) and regularly reviewed. High doses for more than 3 months without any improvement should be discontinued.

6.36 How can I stop myself putting on weight if my medication makes me feel hungry?

A problem with both the typical and atypical antipsychotics – in particular several of the latter – is some patients' experience of feeling more hungry. Some patients even find that they develop a craving for certain foods, especially sweets or carbohydrates. Weight increase is compounded by reduced physical activity, particularly if they are being looked after on a hospital ward. The ready availability of sweet drinks and foods with a lot of sugar in, for example breakfast cereals and frozen pizzas, makes it very easy to put on weight quickly. Controlling your appetite can involve a number of careful steps:

1. Think about what you eat and drink, and try to avoid things with sugar in. Thus, diet brands of cola drinks and/or unsweetened orange juice are good substitutes.
2. Try to eat regular meals, avoiding extra snacks, particularly late at night. Keeping a food diary can help you to see how much you really are eating. You have to be honest of course, putting down everything – even the odd packet of crisps – that you eat in the course of a day.
3. Reducing how much you eat can be helped by having a drink, for example a glass of water, before eating. This gives a sense of fullness without actually putting on calories.
4. Eat as many fruits and vegetables as you want rather than too much heavy pasta and sweet puddings.
5. Eating sometimes comes out of being bored so try to keep busy and, of course, physically active. Exercise won't necessarily make you lose weight, but it will make your body's metabolism increase, making it possible to eat more food without putting on weight.
6. Once you have got into the habit of avoiding sugar, eating regular meals and so forth, you can of course give yourself occasional treats. Break the rules once a week or once a fortnight, and don't try to lose weight too quickly. It is better to adapt slowly, over months, rather than suddenly lose weight (and put it back on again) in the space of several weeks.

Management of schizophrenia: social and psychological treatment

7.1   Is drug treatment alone usually sufficient for most patients with schizophrenia?

Although drug treatment is the essence of modern treatment, and without it the great majority of people would relapse, it is generally accepted that a biopsychosocial approach is the basis of good practice. Medication allows the more florid symptoms, for example intrusive hallucinations or the confusions of thought disorder, to be rolled back, so enabling personal contact. Nurses and doctors can communicate, social programmes can get going, and, for those with sufficient insight, cognitive approaches might even be undertaken. Whether managing acute illnesses – in an emergency setting or on an acute psychiatric ward – caring for people at home or developing rehabilitation programmes, there are certain psychosocial tasks that need completing. Explaining the illness, helping patients to deal with practical and social situations, such as benefit forms or going shopping, and initiating a range of occupational and creative therapies, all are part of modern treatment.

A physical analogy might be the treatment required for a broken leg. Operating on and pinning the broken bones makes it possible for the patient to start moving and walking, but help with dressing, feeding, physiotherapy and relearning how to balance are just as vital in rehabilitation.

7.2   Is counselling helpful or effective in schizophrenia?

The term 'counselling' covers a range of approaches and a range of specialists. There is no evidence that talking to someone about their problems, reflecting back on these problems or even simply listening helps with the active symptoms of schizophrenia. Patients with schizophrenia often cannot communicate properly because of their thought disorder, delusional beliefs or other intrusive experiences. There may be popular notions that counselling can help, and a sympathetic ear is of course generally helpful for most people, whatever their problem, but it is not effective, in terms of evidence-based treatment, for reducing the key handicaps of schizophrenia.

Given the range of clientele that counsellors see, the most important training point, however, is that they learn to recognize the symptoms and pass people on for appropriate treatment. In this sense, counselling can be very helpful in terms of identifying what the problem is and helping patients understand this. Furthermore, once the symptoms have improved, a sensitive counsellor able to talk through fears and problems created by the illness can be much appreciated and very helpful.

7.3 Is there any role for group or marital therapy in the management of schizophrenia?

As with counselling, formal studies of group or marital therapy do not show any specific benefit in improving the symptoms of schizophrenia. There are, however, more structured psycho-educational programmes for the family that can be of benefit. It is, by and large, very difficult for patients with schizophrenia to attend a group given their personal symptoms, at least in the active phase. There may be benefits for those who have recovered and who wish to explore the nature of their experiences, develop social confidence and move on to an understanding of how they can communicate better with others. Likewise, with marital therapy, involving spouses in a treatment programme, identifying and explaining symptoms, and helping them with the burden of care can be a significant aspect of improving outcome. In a formal sense, however, this is not technically 'marital therapy'.

7.4 Can family therapy be helpful in understanding or treating schizophrenia?

There is very good evidence that structured family programmes, based on a psycho-educational approach, can prevent *relapse* in schizophrenic illnesses. The core concept is that of 'expressed emotion' (EE), a measurement of which has been developed in formal research programmes over the past 20 years (*Box 7.1*). Families producing high EE scores seem to generate relapse much more readily than those with low EE scores. In this context, EE is a combination of critical comments, degrees of 'hostility' and emotional over-involvement, some families being so anxious that they end up literally driving their schizophrenic relative into a relapse. Programmes that successfully lower EE lead to much reduced levels of relapse, enhance the family's sense that they can cope with the illness and lower the anxiety levels of vulnerable patients with schizophrenia.

The basis of this approach lies in the difficulty that patients have in dealing with an aroused emotional environment. It is as if they lack a kind of psychological skin, taking on board whatever the worries, moods or concerns are of those around them. Enabling families to reduce this over-anxious atmosphere, even, for example, by reducing face-to-face contact (ensuring that the patient goes to a day centre during the day) is one of the most effective psychosocial treatments available. The relapse rate can be reduced from 70% to 30% by changing the EE from high to low.

BOX 7.1 Expressed emotion and family management

This concept derives from work in the 1950s and 60s on discharged asylum patients, showing that some families seemed to do very badly in caring for relatives with schizophrenia. Nowadays, a standardized assessment, the Camberwell Family Interview, rated from audiotapes, is used to designate an expressed emotion (EE) score, based on:

critical comments:	the number of disapproving or resentful statements, as well as those critical in tone
hostility:	personal criticism, excessive and persistently repeated
emotional over-involvement:	showing excessive worry, over-protectiveness or over-intrusiveness

High scores tend to lead to 50% of patients, and low scores to only about 20%, relapsing within about a year. Taking medication reduces the relapse rate in both groups.

EE may fluctuate, is certainly linked to relatives' feeling more distressed and carrying a higher burden of care, and is valid across most cultures. High-EE family members are more unpredictable in reacting to their relatives' symptoms and are less positive and less 'warm'. Family management aimed at reducing EE, among other problems:

requires specific supervised training in skilled interventions
involves concomitant education on schizophrenia and its symptoms
should focus on the family's problems, as raised by them, with a positive attitude towards the family
can be helped by individual patient sessions and an accompanying carers' support group
may need to continue over several years, to enable patient and family to develop realistic expectations and attitudes.

7.5 Isn't it true that, in the end, individual psychoanalysis is the only real treatment for serious schizophrenia?

There is, perhaps unfortunately, no evidence that insight-orientated, one-to-one (individual) psychoanalysis – along formal Freudian lines, for example – is an effective therapy for schizophrenia. It is often assumed that, if only the resources were available, this kind of in-depth treatment could somehow help those with a serious mental illness, but this is simply not true. Personal psychoanalysis may be helpful for a number of other problems, related to one's upbringing, personality or some forms of depression or anxiety, but it has no particular role in the treatment of schizophrenic symptoms. Some individuals have of course benefited from a personal analysis, alongside, for example, regular treatment with medication, but such outcomes tend to be the exception rather than the rule.

This is not, however, to say that psychiatrists have not tried such an approach. There has certainly been much work and research down the years, since Carl Jung's initial attempts in the early 1900s, to help schizophrenic patients via a psychoanalytic treatment approach (including extensive word association tests), but the results have essentially been disappointing.

7.6 How effective is cognitive-behavioural therapy in the management of schizophrenia?

Cognitive-behavioural therapy (CBT) is one of the more exciting new approaches to the management of schizophrenic illnesses. A number of studies over the past decade have shown considerable benefits, in terms of improved insight, a reduction in the intensity of symptoms, and improved social stability. There has been a debate, however, over how many 'sessions' are needed – a session usually being about 45 minutes to an hour – and about the indicators for successful treatment.

In terms of the latter, the patient clearly has to be prepared to partake in the treatment, but all studies show that up to a third or more 'drop out' quite quickly. Those who do persist seem to show a significant response, often noticeable after only one or two sessions. Some have argued that it is essentially a compliance enhancer in that patients take their medication more regularly (after the cognitive approach) and that is what keeps them well. Others have suggested that there is a specific benefit in developing an insight into one's symptoms, being able to rationalize them, and, essentially, put them out of the front of one's mind. Depending on which studies one accepts, between 20% and 50% of patients show some degree of improvement. See *Box 7.2* for details of the CBT approach, and *Case vignette 7.1*.

CASE VIGNETTE 7.1

A 42-year-old woman with a 10-year-old daughter, whose husband had left her because of his unwillingness to accept her illness, had suffered from schizophrenia for over 15 years. She was tormented by persistent hallucinations, both auditory and olfactory (smells from behind the wall), and was extremely fearful about going outside. Concerns were expressed about the daughter's behaviour, and the nature of the child's living environment was thought to be most unusual. Continual concerns were expressed by the GP, but the patient was unwilling to see a community psychiatric nurse on a regular basis. She regularly complained, after a few sessions with a new nurse, that the nurse was causing aspects of her symptoms. She was willing to accept regular medication and was

---

BOX 7.2 Cognitive-behavioural therapy in schizophrenia

Cognitive-behavioural therapy is aimed at reducing the impact, in particular of delusions and hallucinations, on the patient's behaviour and sense of distress. Approaches include:

For delusions:

1. *Identify automatic thoughts*
   This involves helping patients to understand how they make sense of particular experiences by making automatic assumptions (e.g. 'That person is looking at me intently; therefore he is a threat') and trying to help them to consider alternative reactions (e.g. 'He's looking at me but some people just do that and are quite harmless').

2. *Belief modification*
   Patients are asked – in a non-challenging way – to think of arguments both for and against their beliefs, via what has been termed 'critical collaborative analysis', i.e. 'Let's see if we can work this problem out together.'

3. *Enhancing natural coping strategies*
   Distraction, for example watching television or listening to music, self-relaxation via teaching anxiety management techniques, and taking specific medications are all encouraged

For hallucinations:

1. *Identifying precipitating and relieving factors*
   These may include time of day (voices often being worse at night), certain drugs, certain social situations and states of anxiety. Avoiding such situations, and self-relaxation, can be of significant benefit.

2. *Enhancing natural coping strategies*
   Talking to yourself (or into a mobile telephone!), playing (loud) music, counting under your breath, using ear plugs and taking medication are all useful approaches.

3. *Distraction techniques*
   Changing one's activity, e.g. watching television or talking to someone, concentrating on a task, going to sleep or using a personal cassette player can all be helpful in making voices less intrusive.

---

able to care for herself and her daughter satisfactorily, but had very little social contact with other people because of her fears.

After much persuasion, this lady agreed to accept the offer of a psychological assessment, and a cognitively based approach was undertaken by an experienced clinical psychologist. Although the woman continued to experience hallucinations in two modalities and to express a number of delusional beliefs about the world in which she lived, her ability to talk through these experiences in the CBT sessions was beneficial. Her symptoms persisted, but she was able to develop insight into the fact that other people did not experience them, became less anxious and depressed about her surroundings, and improved her care of her child. Over the course of some 30 sessions, she also agreed to take alternative, atypical medications, which led to an improvement in her personal appearance and better symptom control.

The clinical psychologist eventually left his post, and there were concerns that she would relapse once more in terms of her social behaviour and childcare. However, the gains made in terms of insight, and in terms of her ability to ignore some of her experiences (i.e. to 'park' the voices to the side) persisted. The improved behaviour of her daughter at school was also maintained.

7.7 Can education on the illness help in managing schizophrenia?

There is some evidence that psycho-education for the whole family can reduce the burden of care, enhance the attitudes of families and reduce the rate of relapse in patients with schizophrenia. This approach essentially involves teaching people about the nature of the illness and its symptoms, how these have an effect on their behaviour and how their own reactions can, to some extent, minimize the symptoms. The search continues into the most appropriate psychosocial interventions in terms of the education required, who should deliver it and the training needed. A range of educational materials is being developed countrywide to help to deliver such programmes. These include videos, booklets, tapes and magazines designed to improve knowledge and insight (*see Appendix 2* for details).

7.8 What is the best way of getting the family involved in caring for their relative?

There are several approaches to involving the family in caring for, for example, a 20-year-old man (son, brother, husband) with schizophrenia. Perhaps the most important aspect is explaining the nature of the illness in language that is understandable to the family in terms of their social, cultural and intellectual perspectives. This can be allied to practical tasks, for example helping patients with their shopping, encouraging them to dress and wash appropriately, and supporting them in activities such as going to the day centre. A family-based approach involving family meetings, the use of home rather than hospital treatment and the ready availability of support is of the essence.

Many families feel quite helpless, convinced that their sick relatives will end up in an asylum for the rest of their lives. They also feel scared by the stigma attached to mental illness and perhaps by articles they have read in the local newspaper. Ensuring that the family continue to know about the symptoms, a clear description of the medication and its effects and side-effects, and, if necessary, individual work with family members can all be of benefit. Simple problem-solving techniques can help to identify what the problem is, work out possible solutions and help to select the best one available.

7.9 What is meant by high 'expressed emotion' (see Box 7.1)?

The term 'expressed emotion' (EE) derives from family-based research over the past 40 years.[15] This has clearly shown that families with a high relapse rate (in contrast to those with a low relapse rate) seem to be easily aroused, often critical and/or especially 'anxious' about their schizophrenic relative. Research in this area has shown that one can measure EE, that high EE is deleterious to psychological stability and that lowering it can help patients and families out of difficult circumstances.

7.10 Is living with, and being cared for at home by, their family always best for vulnerable patients?

The simple answer here is 'usually, but not necessarily'. This will of course depend on patients' own attributes, the nature of their parents and the expectations engendered by their social environment. Practical factors such as living space and family finances also play a part.

Much will depend on the nature of patients' particular symptoms – for example, are they noisy at night, shouting at voices? – how they cope with them, the responses of other members of the family and the sheer time involved. By and large, most families want to help care for their relatives, if they are not put at risk, and would like someone to be around on a regular basis to talk to, urgently or as required, in order to maintain stability. Home treatment programmes are generally viewed in a very positive light by both patients and families. The potential and problems of home treatment are outlined in Box 7.3.

7.11 What is the best form of day care treatment?

There is no 'best' form of day care treatment, but a number of individuals respond very well to a daily regime of structured activities and even a degree of part-time work. This is effective both in removing patients from the environment of an anxious (high-EE) parent or family, and in enabling them to develop a sense of achievement in carrying out tasks and being a 'normal' member of working society. A number of families may, however, be resistant to or anxious about this, and it is important to engage them on a step-wise basis.

There is also no specific 'best' approach as different individuals will benefit from different programmes. Some day centres are open 7 days a week, including Sundays and early evenings, and are often run under a

BOX 7.3 Home treatment for schizophrenia

Possible

Home available
Supportive, coping, family
Willing to take medication
No at-risk behaviour or hostile attitudes
Not requiring use of the Mental Health Act
Effective staff and treatment approach available

Unlikely

'No fixed abode'/squatting/homeless
Hostile/unsupportive/uncoping family
Refusing medication
At-risk behaviours, especially if targeted at a family member
Requiring treatment under the Mental Health Act
No suitable staff or treatment time available

'clubhouse' arrangement whereby ex-patients take the lead. Other centres are more structured, run by social services or voluntary groups, and their role will again vary from group to group. Some patients enjoy structured time (e.g. painting and decorating), whereas others are highly resentful about being forced into taking up tasks. Providing a ready-made social network and various leisure activities for those with little money and impaired social skills can lead to friendships, adult education and a truly improved quality of life. The essence of rehabilitation is to be able to judge an individual's needs and potentials, and to concentrate on recreation and occupation that is not too demanding.

7.12 Is it sometimes helpful to keep families and patients apart?

This is certainly true in that a number of patients react badly to their families because of high EE, previous arguments, or disagreements about their current symptoms, dependence and need for medication. It is, by and large, better for younger folk to stay with their families, but it may be better to try those who are older and suffering from chronic symptoms in independent living.

The reason for this is twofold. On the one hand, it is important for schizophrenic patients to keep in touch with their peer group in terms of university, college or training posts. Second, there is in families often a 'gap' between who is doing the caring, who is asking the questions and who is criticizing the unwell family member. Keeping families and patients apart may involve the use of day centres, judicious work schedules and an understanding that improved family behaviour might be of some benefit. Elderly mothers, for example, may be haunted by the worry of who will do the caring after their death, and relieving them of this anxiety can be positive for both mother and patient.

7.13 Can parents or families benefit from individual psychotherapy themselves?

There is no evidence that individual therapy, aimed at just the parents (without the schizophrenic relative) or other family members, is of particular benefit. Such meetings may be comforting and may help one to understand, clarify and respond to difficult demands. As yet though, no formal treatment approaches of this type have been shown to be more beneficial than others in terms of evidence-based practice. Many carers do, however, benefit from carer support groups or more formal psycho-education to help them to understand and cope with the illness.

7.14 What is meant by 'rehabilitation'?

This is the process, using a range of modelling, behavioural and now cognitive techniques, whereby patients with chronic illnesses are helped to return to a degree of independent living. Such programmes are tailored to the individual, particular disabilities being assessed and targeted. Likewise, any skills or strengths are encouraged and worked on, with the aim of gradually replacing the disabilities. Getting patients to dress appropriately, wash regularly and carry out basic tasks such as cooking and cleaning are normally part of the programme, and both residential and day units can be used depending on the level of disability.

Rehabilitation units were classically set up as part of the drive to move people out of asylum hospitals and into the community. Specialist teams consisting of nurses, occupational therapists and psychologists became particularly adept at getting patients to move from states of almost shuffling dependency to relatively independent living. Modern rehabilitation often takes place in community settings, in the patient's own home, in residential homes or in day centres. It aims to improve people's social and personal skills over a number of years while retaining psychological stability (and using medications sensibly). The specialists involved often deal with some of the most difficult, chronic, patients of all, and considerable patience and persistence is required to carry through programmes that may take a number of years.

7.15 How can occupational therapy help someone who has schizophrenia?

A standard form of assessment that patients with schizophrenia undergo when admitted to hospital is an Assessment of Daily Living (ADL). This should be carried out by a trained occupational therapist who will assess how a patient carries out a series of tasks, for example selecting foods and buying them from a shop, preparing them and making a meal. By breaking down these tasks into their smaller components (e.g. safely lighting a gas oven and selecting the right cooking implements), it is possible to analyse and enhance the patient's skills by teaching them (or demonstrating) specific aspects of the whole. Apart from such assessments, occupational therapists will also attempt to engage patients in a range of structured activities, for example partaking in a group discussing current affairs and newspapers, relaxation sessions, creative arts such as pottery or woodwork, or exploring (this being is a more specialist skill) painting or music. The aim is to provide a structured pattern of activities, such as fill the days of ordinary folk, as well as to train people in self-sufficiency in personal care and social activities.

7.16 What do terms like 'low dependence' and 'high dependence' really mean?

These phrases are typically used in assessing a patient's needs in terms of day-to-day living. Standard assessment scales are often used, for example the Social Behaviour Schedule, which looks at social and conversational skills, habits and manners, and difficulties (e.g. hostility) in these contexts. From such assessments emerge an agreed level of dependence, which essentially describes how much support a patient will need.

Patients living in 'low-dependence' units are largely independent, with perhaps a daily or twice-weekly visit from a support worker or carer to help with tidying, shopping or even just in filling out a form. Those in 'high-dependence' units will probably require 24-hour nursing and care, with staff living in the unit and having overnight cover. Highly dependent patients sometimes require a staff complement of two for every individual, but this is unusual and of course very expensive.

In between these poles lie a range of 'medium-dependence' units, perhaps with day-time staff only providing cover at night if there is a crisis, and patients often carrying out many of the daily living tasks (e.g. cooking and cleaning) with the encouragement and support of staff. Stabilizing schizophrenic patients socially will depend on the accuracy with which they can be found just the right environment, avoiding over-expectation and too much pressure yet not allowing them to slide into doing nothing all day, as in old-fashioned institutions. A nice balance in this respect is often found in boarding-out schemes, patients living with a paid adult foster carer who encourages activities, helps with medication and money, and provides companionship and advice.

7.17 Are there any voluntary organizations that can help with the management of schizophrenia?

In the UK, the two most active voluntary organizations are Rethink (formerly called the National Schizophrenia Fellowship), and SANE, with their telephone helpline 'Saneline'. Their details can be found in *Appendix 2*, and they provide a range of informational leaflets, direct telephone support and advice for both patients and carers. There are also many local organizations, often under the rubric of the patients' charity MIND, which again provide a range of services. These include day centres – often of the 'clubhouse' variety – advice sessions, personal counselling, training programmes (e.g. computer skills) and just general support. Such organizations are often able to bring a personal, local touch to services, adding flexibility to those provided by local authorities, hospitals and community mental health teams.

7.18 Is compliance therapy helpful in getting people to take regular medication?

The details of compliance therapy are summarized in *Box 7.4*. This is a relatively new approach, based on actively discussing problems of medication and continuing treatment with patients, and its principles are very much part of modern psycho-education and insight programmes.

7.19 Can any alternative approaches, such as massage or acupuncture, help?

The role of alternative therapies in the treatment of schizophrenia is unproven. There is unfortunately no evidence that acupuncture, homeopathy or other forms of complementary medicine can reduce the symptoms, which is not to say that they may not be of benefit in relaxing individuals, in making people feel acknowledged and in providing a sense of personal support via the complementary therapist. In this sense, they can be seen as 'add-ons', but it is vital that patients and family do not discontinue their regular medication out of the mistaken belief that a complementary therapy is all that is required. Zealots for such alternative approaches, although advocating their therapies with the best of intentions, can sometimes unwittingly cause relapses by the mistaken optimism engendered.

> ## BOX 7.4 Compliance therapy
>
> **Factors affecting compliance/adherence to medication include:**
> - The Illness – delusions; cognitive impairment, stigma
> - The Person – values/beliefs, insight, intelligence
> - The Treatment– therapeutic trust, effects/side-effects, complexity
>
> **The principles of compliance therapy include:**
> - Reflective and careful listening
> - Explaining 'good' and 'bad' aspects of treatment
> - Demonstrating the discrepancy between present behaviour and broader goals
> - 'Normalizing rationales', e.g. medication is normal for many conditions and people
> - Avoid: preaching, labelling and overt argument
>
> **The compliance therapy approach involves (in approximately 4–10 sessions over up to 12 months):**
> - Review the patient's history and views – acknowledge problems with treatment – link relapse with stopping medication
> - Focus on key symptoms and side-effects – balance pros and cons – accept/predict usual reservations about treatment – push adaptive/flexible attitudes
> - Develop reasons for keeping on medication (friendships, avoiding hospital) – acknowledge the social stigma – promote personal strategies for looking after oneself/independence/self-esteem

7.20 Are there any risks in seeing alternative practitioners?

Readers should be careful of a number of specifically antipsychiatry groups, for example the Scientologists, or those offering alternative therapies and denying that medication is in any way necessary. There are also a whole range of alternative therapists claiming to be able to help patients with schizophrenia, and happy to charge large fees, but the evidence for their genuinely being helpful is extremely limited. Before seeing or paying for an unproven therapist, patients are strongly advised to consult with their GP, their family or an established voluntary organization such as MIND or Rethink.

7.21 What training is required for cognitive or family therapy, for example?

There are now quite specific and detailed training programmes for nurses, psychologists, occupational therapists, social workers and psychiatrists (as well as GPs) in these kinds of specialist approach. They generally involve a mixture of seminar work and carrying out treatments under the trained eye of an established therapist, and the total training time may amount to a number of months or several years depending on how frequently one undertakes it. Day-release courses, for 1 day a week, are not uncommon. Some possible sources for such training are given in *Appendix 2*.

7.22 Is there any reason why psychological approaches cannot be tried in the GP's surgery?

There is no reason at all why simple behavioural or cognitive techniques should not be applied by GPs. Some simple techniques such as the 'paradoxical injunction' – telling a semi-mute and rather non-cooperative teenager *not* to talk, while talking about his or her problems with the mother – can be of immediate practical use. Specific behavioural approaches – for example, getting someone gradually accustomed to whatever they fear, say going out of doors, on a graded basis – can also be applied.

The main dilemma is the time required to carry these through successfully, as well as to monitor approaches in a logical way. A typical course of CBT for someone with schizophrenia will involve about half a dozen to a dozen sessions, of up to an hour each, and may require the patient to do some 'homework' in between. The GP can probably best help by reinforcing such techniques – and knowing about them by liaison with a cognitive therapist – rather than undertaking the whole programme directly.

7.23 Is it realistic to try to get a patient back to work?

This should always be kept in mind as a potential aim, particularly if patients have responded to medication, either in the past or currently. Holding unrealistic aims, however, for someone with long-standing symptoms, especially negative ones, will create more pressures than advantages. Nevertheless, the constant encouragement of work as a potential, emphasizing skills and positives rather than failures, and the sheer financial benefits to everyone involved of obtaining a job, are worth pursuing for many patients. By contrast, adopting a pessimistic stance, however realistic, is hardly going to help the family or social and care workers in their attempts to develop patients' personal and behavioural skills.

7.24 What is meant by the phrase 'a sheltered workshop'?

These units, run by social service departments or voluntary organizations, provide excellent working environments for patients who may have limited time-keeping and attention skills but can nevertheless carry out a range of tasks. Saleable items can be produced, so the organizers clearly need to have good contacts with local businesses and shops, and wages are paid (legally because of the 'therapeutic wage' allowance). Patients can thus enhance their income, enjoy a structured day, meet fellow workers and start to normalize their lives in ways that lead to improved self-esteem and a sense of belonging.

7.25 Does 'rehabilitation' mean having to go into hospital?

The term 'rehabilitation' does not imply some form of long-stay hospital, although rehabilitation is typically carried out in some longer-stay units. It essentially embraces a philosophy of trying to restore people to independent living in as untrammelled a setting as possible. The simple business of visiting people regularly at home and helping them with daily tasks so that they can gradually achieve them for themselves, perhaps over several years, is in itself good rehabilitation. Such approaches can also be undertaken by the relatives or immediate family, with support or even formal instruction from relevant mental health staff (e.g. occupational therapists). Some rehabilitation units may be in hospital grounds, simply because that is where they originally were, but just as many nowadays are in independent units in community settings, whether a quiet backstreet or a busy shopping thoroughfare.

7.26 Can you minimize symptoms by using just social and psychological approaches without medication?

Although it is true that social and psychological approaches, for example lowering the EE in families or ensuring that not too much 'face-to-face' contact takes place, can be of benefit, medication remains the cornerstone of treatment. Likewise, ensuring that a patient lives in a stable environment, not too aroused or too under-stimulated, will maintain stability in both social and personal terms. The essence of the modern management of schizophrenia revolves around the phrase 'biopsychosocial' in that a range of skills, a range of specialists and a range of aims (symptom control, psychological and social stability) are all pursued.

7.27 Are there any particular training courses or types of job that patients with schizophrenia are best at undertaking?

It is difficult to say that one particular job would be perfect for someone with schizophrenia because individuals are so different. If one considers the kinds of problem that patients with schizophrenia have to deal with, for example distraction from intermittent hallucinations or difficulty motivating themselves, work that can take those difficulties on board is most suitable. This would involve flexible hours, tasks that can be broken up into separate components, the ability to take breaks rather than keep working solidly and tasks that will not be too impaired if people are occasionally distracted. There are also a number of patients who find it difficult to deal with the public or large crowds of people but can happily work at a computer or quietly on their own. Environmental stability (and relative quietness), a relatively stable work routine and lack of time pressure are the most important ingredients.

7.28 Can Assertive Outreach Teams really get people better?

Among the newer approaches to the management of schizophrenia are Assertive Outreach Teams (AOTs), initially introduced in the USA. They were very much designed to provide the extra support and help that regular community teams were unable to provide and to address the needs of those who found it hard to engage with services and tended to relapse regularly. AOTs are based around a general philosophy of team involvement (i.e. everyone knowing every patient that the team is looking after), having no more than perhaps 8–12 patients per team member – i.e. a high staff/care ratio – and being able to undertake a range of tasks. These include organizing medication, taking people to their GP, helping to tidy the house, going on visits, filling out welfare benefit forms and delivering more specific therapies such as anger management or anxiety relief.

Table 7.1 summarizes the AOT's role and philosophy. Such teams are seen as an essential component of the National Service Framework and NHS Plan, funding now being provided in every district to set up an appropriate AOT.

TABLE 7.1 Assertive Outreach Team	
Rationale	To provide intensive care and support in the community for patients who frequently relapse, who are at risk to themselves or others and who do not engage with regular services (i.e. GP, outpatient department, community team)
Principles	1. A *multidisciplinary* team of nurses, social workers, psychologists, social therapists and psychologists
	2. High patient/staff ratio – each worker has only 8–12 patients
	3. Based on teamwork – everyone knows about the clientele and helps to solve problems
	4. Rapid response and close, regular contact – building up trust and helping with practical tasks, e.g. shopping/repairs
	5. Aimed at enhancing compliance, problem-solving and avoiding hospitalization
Benefits	Use of hospital beds reduced by approximately 30%
	Usually liked by patients and carers
	Good job satisfaction for team members as is a creative, flexible pattern of working

7.29 What is the effect of Early Intervention and Crisis Response Teams?

Both of these types of team are also part of the NHS Plan, and the government is pledged to providing funding for them. Early Intervention is based upon the prognosis for schizophrenia being strongly related to the length of illness prior to treatment (e.g. *see Box 8.3*). Such teams therefore target younger people with early signs of illness in order to engage them, get them into treatment, help their families and try to minimize the harm produced by prolonged symptoms and the social effects of the illness in itself.

Crisis Response Teams are aimed not specifically at patients with schizophrenia but rather at handling the range of mental health crises that can occur, at home or in community settings, without resorting to hospital admission if at all possible. Such teams will see people at home, deliver a range of home treatment packages, stay with people for much of the day or two or three times a week for 2 or 3 hours, relieve the family and generally provide the kind of intensive support and nursing that would otherwise be available only in hospital. There is evidence in some areas that such teams can reduce the number of beds required for admissions, but the intensive nature of their work needs evaluation. Although often initially staffed by young and enthusiastic individuals, the tone tends to change after a few years. They are certainly popular with patients and families, who feel that their needs are being addressed, but such teams clearly have to be judicious in taking on and moving on from people, and this can lead to complications in their relationship with the regular community mental health teams.

7.30 What does the recent National Institute for Clinical Excellence guideline advise about treatment in primary and secondary care?

This guideline, based on the best evidence available, has emphasized a number of important principles in modern care for schizophrenia. These include ensuring care across all stages and working in partnership with carers and patients, ensuring early referral and intervention by the right types of service (e.g. day hospitals and crisis/home teams), using medications safely and effectively, and promoting recovery.

Factors highlighted include: maintaining optimism; early and easy access to professional help; a comprehensive assessment of social and healthcare needs; providing information and support, and trying to ensure consent to treatment; having consideration for language and culture; and (if appropriate) trying to obtain advance directives. Advance directives are drawn up by patients, their chosen carer (if available) and their nurse, doctor or therapist. The documents outline the treatments patients would prefer to receive if they became so unwell that they could not look after themselves. A signed summary is kept in their notes and regularly updated.

Services outlined by the guideline should include: community mental health teams; inpatient and day patient facilities; crisis and home treatment teams; social and group support; access to a senior psychiatrist (and a second opinion if necessary); use of the Care Programme Approach (CPA) to integrate services; and access to a GP to ensure physical health assessments and maintain support and medication. In terms of *relapse prevention*, the use of AOTs (*see Table 7.1*), CBT and family education, supportive employment programmes and continuing antipsychotic medication (oral or depot) are all integral to improving outcome.

 PATIENT QUESTIONS

7.31   Should every patient now receive CBT?

There is no doubt that many patients can be helped by this approach, in that CBT is a way of dealing with some very bothersome symptoms. If, for example, you are regularly troubled by voices, techniques can be developed for minimizing them, distracting yourself from them or even to some degree getting the voices to be more pleasant and under control. However, not everyone benefits, and it is usually quite clear within one or two sessions whether you yourself will start to feel better. It is most important therefore that any CBT is properly monitored and assessed, otherwise it can go on for month after month and even lead to disappointment. It must be emphasized that this is not really a treatment aimed at eliminating completely your symptoms but it is designed to help you cope with them better and to stop them becoming too much the centre of your life.

7.32   Should all patients really have their own social worker?

Most modern community mental health teams, particularly those involved in caring for patients with schizophrenia, will run on what is called a multidisciplinary basis. That is to say, within a team of 15–20 people, or even more, there will be a number of social workers, community psychiatric nurses, an occupational therapist or two, psychologists, psychiatrists, support workers and administrators. Depending on one's needs, each patient should be allocated what is now called a care coordinator (used to be called a keyworker), whose task is to keep in personal contact with you. This may be a social worker but can just as easily be a community nurse or community support worker.

Although their skills and experience will vary, each team member should be able to carry out, alone or with one of their colleagues, all the work needed to ensure the right sort of care. It is also important to be aware of

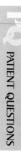

just what the care coordinator – or social worker – actually can and cannot do. Remember, if you have got a housing problem, they have to contact the Housing Department – they are not part of the Housing Department – to try to get things mended, arrange appointments, etc. Likewise, they do not have loads of money that they can dish out at every single crisis. They will do their best to help you in both of these respects – i.e. crises in housing or money – but the whole point of the team is that everyone tries to pull together, contributing their separate skills while attempting to ensure a personal service.

7.33   What is meant by a CPA meeting?

It is now an established part of community care that every patient with support needs – and many people with schizophrenia will need help outside hospital – should be helped via the CPA process. This essentially tries to make sure that all your needs are assessed, that someone is responsible for trying to get particular things done and that someone is checking up on what is going on.

Therefore, when you have a CPA meeting, at home, at a community team base or on a psychiatric ward, it is essentially a means of ensuring that the help you are told you are going to get really will be provided. During the discussion, the care coordinator will try to clarify with you what your needs are, for example in terms of medication, housing, welfare benefits or daytime activities. He or she will then make some suggestions, doctor's appointments will be agreed (if necessary), and someone will take the lead on, for example, introducing you to the day centre or helping you fill out a housing application form. A care plan will be written up, summarizing all this, and often a crisis plan to ensure help in case you start to become unwell. The document should be signed, a further meeting date agreed, to check out what has and has not been done – for example, in 3 months' time – and a further plan drawn up then. This may seem like a lot of paperwork, but it provides a means of reviewing whether or not you are getting the things you need.

CPA meetings can be a little bit ponderous and formal, and many people are rather frightened of them. Remember, they are designed entirely to help you by finding out what *you* need. If things are fairly clear in your mind, the meetings should not last more than a few minutes, but they should help you feel clear on what is being done and what will be done.

7.34   Can someone with schizophrenia be treated against his or her will (*see Table 7.2*)?

Yes. In the UK, the 1983 Mental Health Act provides the rules of involuntary treatment, and every country in the world has some such provision. Because of the need to protect human rights, while at the same time ensuring the right to treatment even though you may be unable to care for yourself, there is also a system of inspecting and reviewing all those 'sectioned' (i.e. detained involuntarily in hospital) under the Act. There is thus a Mental

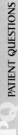

Health Act Commission, and any patient can appeal to a Mental Health Review Tribunal to have an order set aside. As outlined in *Table 7.2*, there are various types of order, varying from brief 'emergency' sections (up to 72 hours) to longer-term treatment orders lasting up to 6 months if necessary.

In terms of the Mental Health Act, 'schizophrenia' comes under the heading of 'mental illness' and has to be serious enough, with risks to health, to warrant detention. Most patients are of course happy to accept treatment voluntarily, and many detained patients are even discharged before the end of a given 'section' once they are well and can accept that they need treatment.

TABLE 7.2 Mental Health Act 1983 – some commonly used sections (England & Wales only)

Section	Purpose	Length (max)	Who recommends?	Who applies
2	Assessment and treatment	28 days	Two doctors, including 1 'approved'*	Approved Social Worker (ASW) or nearest relative
3	Treatment Order	6 months	ASW	ASW
4	Emergency assessment	72 hours	One doctor	ASW
5(2)	Inpatient detention	72 hours	One doctor	–
37	Hospital Order (Court)	6 months	Two doctors (approved)*	The court

*Approved Doctors (under Section 12) are essentially those with special experience and training (i.e. psychiatrists).

N.B. 1: Patients can only be detained if suffering from:
(a) defined mental disorder
and (b) it is of a nature or degree warranting admission to hospital
and (c) for the patient's health or safety, or for the protection of other persons

N.B. 2: 'Mental disorder' includes mental illness, mental impairment and severe mental impairment (i.e. learning difficulty) and psychopathic disorder (i.e. severe personality disorder); it *excludes* promiscuity, sexual deviancy or drug/alcohol dependence

Course and prognosis

8.1 How quickly does a first-onset schizophrenic illness present?

The onset of recognizable schizophrenia usually develops over a matter of weeks or months rather than days. The typical story will be of someone who has *changed*, in terms of what they talk about and what they say, as noted by the family rather more than the patient. Studies have unfortunately shown that the time of first intervention is often more than a year, on average, after the first symptoms, as later reported by the patient. Roughly speaking, therefore, there are three fairly standard types of first onset, namely 'insidious', over a year or two (often of hebephrenic type (*see* Q *1.19*)), 'average', over the course of a few months (usually paranoid type (*see Table 1.4*)), and 'acute'. The latter includes a time of onset of a few days to 3 or 4 weeks but accounts for fewer than 10% of cases.

8.2 Is it common for schizophrenic patients suddenly to become unwell, in a matter of a few days or even hours?

No. The sudden onset of an illness like schizophrenia is unusual, and this type of presentation usually reflects an alternative diagnosis, for example a manic episode, a puerperal illness or possibly a drug-induced disorder. Such acute states should always be carefully reviewed in terms of their possible physical bases, and if this is a 'first-onset' presentation, it is wisest to avoid concluding too readily that it is a form of schizophrenia. Unusual presentations of, for example, meningitis, or even hypoglycaemic attacks, will be part of the differential diagnosis, hence the need for a careful and comprehensive physical and psychiatric assessment.

CASE VIGNETTE 8.1 ACUTE PSYCHOSIS ... SCHIZOPHRENIA, MANIA, OR WHAT?

A 22-year-old student with no previous psychiatric problems was travelling in India with friends. He developed a rather severe form of diarrhoea and vomiting with a high fever (as did a friend), and, over the course of 2 or 3 days, apparently became 'confused'. His friends tried to support him, but he now became rather paranoid and over-active, and fled into the night. Fortunately, he was picked up by the local police and taken to the local mental hospital.

He continued to show signs of over-activity, apparently hallucinating at night and being very restless, intermittently confused over time and place, and expressing unusual ideas. He was treated with haloperidol (one of the few local medications available) and to some degree calmed down. After about 10 days, his father, who had flown out to help to care for the student, was able to fly him back to the UK.

At home in England, the young man continued to exhibit a mixed pattern of symptoms, sometimes manic, sometimes paranoid and required continuing antipsychotic medication as well as benzodiazepines to help with sleep and restlessness. Because of his almost 'driven' state of mental over-alertness, a pragmatic decision was taken to discontinue his antimalarial medication (chloroquine) and within 4 days he had calmed down, as if a switch had been turned off. A review of the Indian medical literature showed many case reports of similar psychotic presentations. Apart from a post-illness depression he remained well, returning to his studies later that year.

A working diagnosis concluded that the young man had had an acute polymorphic psychosis, either as a post-viral reaction or caused by a sensitivity to antimalarial drugs. This was *not* schizophrenia.

8.3 What is the best way of finding out how long someone has been unwell?

This is one of the great dilemmas of modern schizophrenia research. Generally speaking, if patients can give a good history, it is worth asking them when they last felt reasonably well or their normal selves. It is also worth asking them what has happened in their lives over the past year or two (rather than the past few weeks) because that will often give a clue to significant changes taking place. They may thus say that people started treating them badly or teasing them at college, that they started feeling 'depressed' or even that some time ago their drinks were 'spiked'.

The other sources of information are the family or close friends. They will often give a different time course from that offered by the patient, usually (but not necessarily) somewhat longer. They will describe a sense of personality change, for example a degree of social withdrawal ('He just keeps to himself in his room, doctor'), or unusual idiosyncrasies such as constantly washing or making strange signals or gestures. The general rule is that illnesses have usually been going on longer than the overt presentation suggests. There is of course no means of assessing the time course in terms of the specific presenting symptoms, nor do any psychological or biochemical investigations help to clarify matters.

8.4 Can patients really cover up symptoms and stay living at home, or even working, for a year or more?

This is certainly possible since the embarrassments of the symptoms, the fear of being called 'mad' and the sheer reality of the experiences can obscure the diagnosis, for both the patient and family. Patients may, for example, present complaining of being teased or harassed at work in rather non-specific ways that do not stop them carrying on with their work but may have involved a number of reviews and even investigations of a formal nature. In terms of home, young men often, quite naturally, start to develop rather personal lives, refusing to talk to their parents about their relationships or what they are doing; even the most diligent mother or father may thus find it difficult to see anything wrong. The different lifestyles, clothing, personal habits and even language of younger people –

remembering that schizophrenia typically presents in the late teens or early 20s – can sometimes be hard to pathologize. Up to 20% of patients are never really properly diagnosed, and even those who are may merely be seen to have some form of depression or anxiety, or a somewhat shy disposition. It may take quite detailed and even intrusive questioning to clarify an individual patient's experiences.

8.5 Can one predict the outcome from any particular symptom or pattern of symptoms?

It is generally accepted that symptoms in themselves are poorly predictive of any particular outcome. There is, however, a view that positive symptoms (e.g. hallucination and thought broadcast), if apparent early in the illness, should predict a better outcome than the slow onset of predominantly negative symptoms such as apathy or anhedonia. *Table 8.1* attempts to summarize the 'good outcome' and 'bad outcome' scenarios in terms of predicting what might follow. No individual symptom, whether positive or negative, has any significant predictive meaning, the pattern of onset *and* symptoms (especially over the first 2 years) seeming to be most relevant. Many patients will have a mix of indicators, and consistency of treatment may be more important than anything else.

8.6 Does the length of onset in any way predict the response to treatment?

As outlined in *Table 8.1*, a short onset – a matter of days or weeks – is much more likely to lead to a better response to treatment and a better outcome. By contrast, the longer the onset, because of more insidious symptoms, for example over 2 or 3 years, the longer it will take to generate effective treatment. This is one of the few really 'hard' facts known about schizophrenia, derived from a number of studies looking at the course of the illness. Therefore, the importance of early detection, whether at school, at home or in the workplace, alongside continuing attempts at removing stigma, cannot be underestimated.

8.7 Is there a typical course of the illness?

No, but, rather like multiple sclerosis, several patterns have emerged depending on length of onset, prevalence of positive or negative symptoms, response to treatment and compliance with continued medication. Approximately 60–70% of patients typically respond to initial treatment and return to some significant level of functioning or even to work. Sadly,

TABLE 8.1 Prognostic factors in schizophrenia

	Good outcome	Poor outcome
Onset	Acute (days/weeks)	Insidious (months/years)
Age	Over 30	Adolescent
Gender*	Female	Male*
Family history	Nil (or for affective illness)	Positive for schizophrenia
Social	Working/good social contacts	Isolated/unemployed
	Low family EE	High family EE
Intelligence	Above average	Below average/learning disability
	No cognitive impairment	Cognitive impairment
Symptoms	Mood disturbance	Flat/withdrawn
	Positive	Negative
Investigation (computed tomography brain scan)	No brain abnormalities	Enlarged cerebral ventricles
Drugs/alcohol	Not misusing	Substance misuse
Treatment	Earlier response, without side-effects	Limited/nil response and/or significant side-effects
	Compliant/insightful	Denial of illness/non-compliant
Geography (?)	Developing country	Industrialized country

EE, expressed emotion (*see Box 7.1*)
*This may simply reflect the earlier onset in males

80% or more will relapse over the course of the next 2 or 3 years, and the next recovery may be a little less positive than the first. At this stage, many patients will that accept they need regular treatment, their families will be involved and supportive, and the patients should remain stable. Various typical illness patterns are outlined in *Figure 8.1*.

One group of patients, however, constantly refuse medication, relapse after a while and have a 'revolving door' illness that generally leads to declining personal abilities and even institutionalization. This group accounts for about a third of individuals over the course of 5–10 years. At the other end of the spectrum of course, some 10–20% of patients have only one illness and then stay well, whereas so-called 'late-phase' recovery is seen in over 10% of early non-responders to treatment.

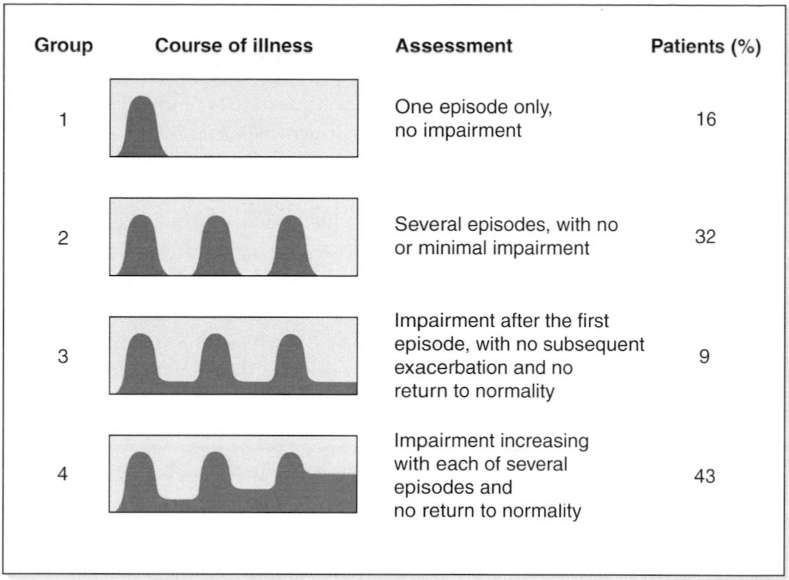

Group	Course of illness	Assessment	Patients (%)
1		One episode only, no impairment	16
2		Several episodes, with no or minimal impairment	32
3		Impairment after the first episode, with no subsequent exacerbation and no return to normality	9
4		Impairment increasing with each of several episodes and no return to normality	43

Fig. 8.1 Graded course of illness for patients with schizophrenia during five years as indicated by episodes of illness, symptomatology and social impairment at assessments (n = 107). From Kerwin R, Travis M 2001 *Managing Relapse in Schizophrenia*. Science Press, London, with permission

8.8 Do younger patients respond better to treatment than older patients?

No. It is generally accepted that the younger the patient, the more likely there will be a more chronic outcome. Patients who become ill in their mid-teens, for example, often with a mixture of positive and negative symptoms – outlined under the 'hebephrenic' label (*see* Q 1.19) – are those who will need to be most closely reviewed and supported. By contrast, if the illness does not come on until the late 20s or early 30s, patients will have developed a personality, possibly settled down and had a family, and should have developed a career; the outcome in psychosocial terms is clearly going to be better. This reflects why women often do so much better than men, their illnesses typically coming on 4 or 5 years later.

8.9 Why are the more chronic patients usually male?

Chronicity in schizophrenia is associated with negative symptoms and early onset. The latter in particular is associated with the male gender, the average age of onset being around 22–23 years, by contrast with 27–28 years for females. This in itself would generate more chronicity, but there seem to be other aspects of being male that do not go well with suffering from schizophrenia. These include the need for higher doses of medication (with concomitant side-effects), a greater impairment of social role (i.e. not being able to go out and work to feed a family), the greater likelihood of drug and/or alcohol abuse and a tendency to reduced compliance with taking medication. This may be associated with the significant (but often not reported, perhaps out of embarrassment) sexual side-effects suffered by many male patients, in particular erectile failure and delayed or absent ejaculation.

The consequence of all this is that male patients with a chronic illness are much more prevalent (by about 60% or 65%) than females in rehabilitation or institutional settings.

8.10 Does early treatment help with the long-term outcome?

Early treatment is generally accepted as the gold standard to which we should all be aiming in the management of schizophrenia. There is evidence from a number of studies that the more quickly the treatment is initiated, the better the long-term outcome, although outcome is difficult to measure. The fact that people actually receive treatment has in itself nowadays led to the disappearance of the chronic, self-neglecting, often mute and doubly incontinent patients who infested the back wards of the old asylums. Although early treatment is associated with both a better response to treatment and a reduction in subsequent, persisting, symptoms, even on relapse, this does not, however, seem to prevent relapse.

Some possible outcome measures are outlined in *Table 8.2*, illustrating the dilemma of what 'outcome' really means and how we can evaluate the effects of treatment.

TABLE 8.2 Possible outcome measures in schizophrenia

Symptoms	Positive/negative ⎫ Persisting, many or few? mood-related ⎭
Course of illness	Relapsing/remitting – how many times?
Development of cognitive impairments	How measured? IQ tests or sub-tests?
Social network	How many friends, contacts, activities?
Quality of life	Subjective satisfaction, income, drugs?
Violence	Episodes of aggression, suicide attempts, law-breaking?
Daily life	Work, housing, family?

8.11 What is meant by the term 'chronic schizophrenia'?

This somewhat denigratory term outlines a group of patients who have continued to suffer from active symptoms of the illness over a number of years (*Fig. 8.2*). Such an outcome usually occurs despite a range of medications taken at up to full dosage and despite receiving full inpatient rehabilitation programmes. Patients should have been ill for at least 2 if not 5 years to qualify as 'chronic' and will show a number of personal deficits in terms of their limited self-care, a degree of social withdrawal and an increasing number of neurological symptoms (for example, abnormal mouth or body movements). Depending on the level of severity, such patients with persisting symptoms of some sort constitute 30–50% of schizophrenia in general.

In *ICD-10*[4], category F20.5 is entitled 'residual schizophrenia'. This is seen as a chronic stage in the development of the disorder, with prominent negative symptoms, clear evidence of a previous psychotic episode (meeting the criteria for schizophrenia), at least a year of substantially reduced chronic positive symptoms such as delusions, and the absence of dementia or any other brain disease. Such patients generally come under the care of rehabilitation specialists and continuing care rehabilitation teams.

8.12 Do some patients just inevitably go down hill?

Although this is not a common course (*see Q. 8.7* and *8.11*), a downhill decline is certainly seen in a few patients. This is most distressing to watch as it will generally involve self-neglect, positive symptoms such as paranoid beliefs and hallucinations, being resistant to continued treatment (partly because of non-compliance), a varying degree of cognitive impairment (*Box 8.1*) and increasing social neglect on the part of other people. Such 'malignant' cases are well known, and some individuals seem to deteriorate very quickly over the course of 3 or 4 years, even as young people (e.g. in their 20s and 30s). The reasons for this are uncertain and may reflect different underlying pathologies.

8.13 Are schizophrenic patients more prone to any other regular illnesses?

In terms of associations with the illnesses themselves, there is no clear-cut evidence that schizophrenia is regularly associated with other physical conditions, apart from diabetes. There are of course the secondary effects of being overweight, of excessive smoking and of being unfit. Enhanced

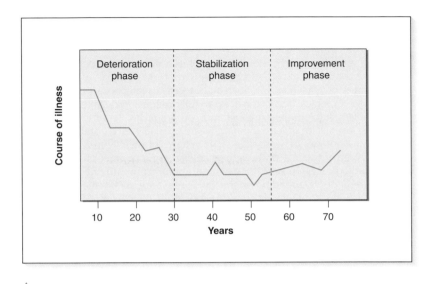

Fig. 8.2 Model of the course of illness of chronic schizophrenia. From Kerwin R, Travis M 2001 *Managing Relapse in Schizophrenia*. Science Press, London, with permission

BOX 8.1 Cognitive impairment in schizophrenia

■ Some degree of cognitive impairment is noted in up to 85% of patients when comprehensively assessed by formal methods

■ It is common to encounter various forms of memory impairment (e.g. semantic and episodic memory)

■ The frontal lobe 'executive function' (e.g. organizing a complex series of tasks) is often found to be impaired

■ Cognitive impairment is *not* improved by conventional antipsychotic agents* but tends to influence long-term outcome more than the symptoms do

■ There is no correlation between cognitive impairment and specific symptoms, although it is more often associated with negative symptoms

■ Rehabilitation can improve task performance (e.g. via incentives or practice), but there is often little gain in overall functioning

*The effect of atypical medication remains unclear

cardiovascular difficulties, therefore, and forms of breathing difficulty associated with chronic airways disease (e.g. bronchitis) are the main associated medical problems. It should also be remembered that patients with schizophrenia are much more likely to have bouts of depression, are more likely to be using drugs (usually soft drugs such as cannabis) and may be more prone to a range of accidents. Schizophrenia is thus associated with an excess mortality deriving from the risks of suicide (about 10% of patients), other violent deaths and physical illness.

8.14 Does smoking cannabis significantly affect the outcome?

There has been a furious debate in the national press, as well as in the specialist psychiatric press, over the role of cannabis, or its constituent ingredient tetrahydrocannabinol, on an individual's mental state (*see Table 4.2*). There is certainly evidence that if one suffers from schizophrenia, smoking cannabis can bring on more acute symptoms, although these will often resolve quite quickly. There is also evidence that a number of patients continue to smoke cannabis in various forms throughout their 'illness careers'. A limited amount of evidence has shown that early use of cannabis is associated with impaired outcome in long-term schizophrenia, but whether this is cause or effect remains debatable.

8.15 If there is a 'dual diagnosis', and patients also have problems with drugs or alcohol, does that affect the prognosis?

There is clear evidence from studies on dual diagnosis (*Box 8.2*) that up to 50% of patients, particularly in inner cities or other deprived areas, have a significant dependence on other drugs, for example heroin, crack cocaine and alcohol. Such complications will clearly affect the prognosis because of the high rate of relapse, the higher doses of medication that may be needed, and the risk to the individual of being both alcohol dependent (with its effects on the liver) and a whole range of physical disorders. The constant use of illicit supplies of opiates or cocaine creates significant health risks (e.g. HIV) as well as impoverishment and dangerous contacts with exploitative criminals.

There has been recent guidance from the Department of Health on the management of people with dual diagnosis problems as there is a worsening of the prognosis if someone with schizophrenia has, for example, a significant alcohol dependence. This can lead to exploitation, self-neglect and marginalization in terms of social contacts.

BOX 8.2 Dual diagnosis

■ This commonly refers to schizophrenia *and* substance misuse affecting one patient
■ The co-morbidity of schizophrenia (e.g. with learning difficulty or diabetes) is also sometimes termed a 'dual diagnosis'
■ Between 30% and 50% of patients have significant substance misuse (especially of alcohol, cannabis or cocaine, e.g. crack)
■ Reasons for substance misuse include:
   – Anxiety relief, mood elevation and pleasure
   – Self-medication for symptoms or side-effects
   – Peer group or 'dealer' pressures (e.g. exploitation of vulnerable people)
   – Help with sleep, 'pain' and low self-esteem
■ Treatment may require:
   – Hospital admission – to review medication and/or symptoms; withdrawal (detoxification); plan of support and aftercare
   – Specialist dual diagnosis team or community psychiatric nurse/support worker
   – Psycho-education for the patient/family with planned rehousing or day care
   – A four-phase approach – engagement; persuasion; active treatment (i.e. substitutes, skills training and support); relapse prevention

8.16 Can families help in the more chronic illnesses?

Yes. There is now a greatly increased understanding of how patients who seem to have chronic schizophrenic illnesses respond to family input. This can help via family or group psycho-education, or with more formal approaches to lower the 'expressed emotion' (*see Box 7.1*) that often leads to relapse. Degrees of contact between a patient and family members, appropriate daytime activity and trying to remain calm and relaxed when talking to someone with schizophrenia are all part of a supportive approach. By contrast, the lack of any available family is a significant problem – especially in inner city areas – when dealing with people with high dependence needs. It is well understood that families are often the lynchpin of care for a range of illnesses of the 'minor' neurotic type, but the more chronic problems of regular schizophrenia are often minimized in the right kind of friendly, supportive family home.

8.17 Are patients with schizophrenia more prone to dementia or other brain diseases?

There is no evidence that patients with schizophrenia have a higher rate of vascular or non-vascular dementia. There is also no evidence that they suffer more often from any kind of early-onset neurological disorder, or any specific association with other brain diseases. A range of brain illnesses (e.g. temporal lobe damage and enhanced infections such as encephalitis) can of course in themselves lead to schizophrenia-like symptoms, as can severe fevers in the vulnerable. It is also well known that various neurological 'soft signs' (e.g. dyspraxia) are commonly seen, as are various involuntary movements (e.g. tics, and grimaces) that may be exacerbated by medication, leading to 'tardive' dyskinesia (*see Q. 5.18*).

8.18 In the long term, what proportion of patients do quite well and live independently?

The standard figures for long-term follow-up are roughly as follows:

- Approximately 20–30% of patients live independently, or almost independently, in the community, some of them with jobs.
- About 40% of patients live in varying degrees of dependence, either with families or in hostels, a few of them holding down 'sheltered workplace' jobs but being supported in terms of day centres or nursing/social care input.
- Some 30% require institutional care of varying degrees of complexity or even security. Such patients are usually not capable of independent living.

8.19 Do any personality factors affect the outcome?

There is an association between schizotypal disorder and schizophrenia in terms of the former's social withdrawal, rather idiosyncratic beliefs and impaired social contact. No other specific personality factors have been associated with schizophrenia in anecdotal comment, formal research or computerized analyses of detailed histories. Some patients with schizophrenia (about 1% on current ratings) will, however, also have a number of personality problems, and this combination can be quite troublesome.

The dilemma of feeling rather paranoid and 'got at' alongside limited impulse control is particularly dangerous. Any aspects of the paranoid or dissocial types of personality disorder, or even what is called 'emotionally unstable personality disorder' (but more usually described as 'borderline disorder'), are all likely to lead to refusal to take medication, lack of insight into the illness and a more chronic illness course. The difficulty in distinguishing between personality disorder and schizophrenia in some patients makes for even greater difficulties in caring for them.

8.20 Is life expectancy reduced in patients with schizophrenia?

It certainly seems to be, mainly because of the physical effects of excessive smoking, lack of exercise, being overweight and the general self-neglect that many patients with schizophrenia adopt towards their health. It is very difficult to get exact figures for this. Roughly speaking, life expectancy will be reduced by about 10–15%, key factors being, for example, the number of cigarettes inhaled (*see Q. 8.13*).

8.21 Can the newer drug treatments affect the long-term outcome?

We do not know the answer to this yet because atypicals have been around only since the early 1990s. It may be that over the course of prolonged treatment – for example 10–20 years – problems will emerge that are similar to those seen with dopamine blockers. There is, however, evidence that symptoms of tardive dyskinesia – mouth movements, jerky body movements and shaking hands – can be improved in those taking clozapine, and there is already evidence that long-term outcome is much better than it was before drug therapy became available.

The main hopes for the newer 'atypical' forms of drug treatment centre around improved compliance, the loss of movement disorder side-effects (e.g. akathisia) and reduced impairment in terms of, for example, sexual dysfunction. It nevertheless seems quite clear that, despite much intensive research, the long-term outcome of patients on some of the newer drug treatments has yet to be established (*see Box 9.1*).

8.22 If there is a known cause, might that have an impact on the prognosis?

This is most unlikely. Not only is the cause of schizophrenia not known in general, but it is also very unusual that a particular person is felt to have the illness because of a known, definite, causative factor. Even were that so, a corroborative history would probably establish other factors prior to the 'apparent' key factor. Nevertheless, many patients and families attribute the illness to some specific event (e.g. bereavement) or personal stressor. This 'search after meaning' is understandable but not usually very helpful in treatment terms. Blaming parents, for example, is quite common, but the outcome will be enhanced only in a non-critical family environment! (and methods of child-rearing have *no* aetiological role).

Someone with a known illness – for example, a head injury – that can be repaired is clearly likely to have a much more stable lifestyle anyway, and symptoms are generally much fewer and more circumscribed.

8.23 What happened to patients before the availability of modern drug treatments?

The main recourse for patients with ongoing schizophrenia prior to the new treatments of the modern drug era was 'the asylum', renamed 'the mental hospital' in 1930. Here, patients with schizophrenia in particular were carefully stored in increasingly large institutions up to 3000 or more strong. Some drugs, for example forms of barbiturate, were used to try to sedate individuals. Also employed were electroconvulsive therapy, straitjackets, enclosed hot baths (to calm patients down) and a range of other desperate remedies, such as lobotomy.

Whatever the minor difficulties now experienced by many patients, in terms of weight gain for example, the comparison to the state of patients before the availability of any medication is striking. Any attempt to reproduce such conditions as they lived in would be ethically unjustified, even though the experimental, drug-free 'Villa 21' at Shenley Hospital, run by Dr David Cooper (an acolyte of Dr R.D. Laing) remains quite famous in modern studies. In essence, a patient unable to accept modern drug treatment would be at significant risk of self-harm, neglect and a life dominated by a range of unpleasant symptoms such as hallucinations.

8.24 Can the environment – urban or rural, European or tropical – affect the outcome?

Research generally seems to show that rural, non-European (i.e. Third World) environments are better for patients with schizophrenia in terms of their social recovery.[1] This is one of the most intriguing findings of the past 20 or 30 years and is not fully understood. It is thought to be partly because urban environments such as London (especially the inner boroughs) attract a range of chronic patients who have drifted in from elsewhere looking for cheap housing and/or relatively accessible support. Furthermore, the '9 to 5' working environment in which many people find themselves militates against convalescing and developing confidence. Studies show that 45% of schizophrenic patients in developing countries are seen to be recovered after 5 years, compared with 25% in developed countries, whereas 75% of the former are minimally impaired compared with only 33% of the latter.

Part of what this difference tells us is that the skills required to negotiate the modern world are often outside those of patients with chronic schizophrenia. A supportive environment with a range of activities suited to patients' needs (and speed) is often the key priority.

8.25 What are the best predictors of a good outcome?

This is summarized in *Table 8.1* above, but in essence a good outcome is associated with positive symptoms, a relatively brief onset, a degree of intelligence and good family support. The opposite applies to the predictors of a poor outcome.

8.26 How serious is the risk of suicide in schizophrenia?

There is unfortunately a genuine risk of both self-harm and suicide in patients with schizophrenia. Figures vary, depending on the age groups studied and the countries in which the studies take place. The definition of suicide in itself – for example, the 'open' verdict when how someone died is genuinely uncertain – further complicates the issue. The most pessimistic figures are around 10–15% of all those suffering from the illness in the course of their lifetime, but this is often compounded by being combined with personality problems, very difficult personal circumstances and drug or alcohol dependence.

There is no doubt, however, that some people are profoundly affected by both the symptoms of schizophrenia and their despair at having such an illness. In the early days, symptoms of depression, as well as, for example, threatening voices, can so drive individuals to distraction that they really think that life is not worthwhile. Patients are also prone to sudden impulsive acts, caused by beliefs, for example, that their bodies are infected or that something has to be cut out, or by the sheer physical discomfort, even pain, of their somatic sensations. Preventing suicide, in terms of early diagnosis, counteracting stigma and providing supportive personal care, is integral to good quality management.

Of interest is a recent series of studies (*see the references*) suggesting that clozapine can genuinely reduce suicidal outcome in patients with difficult schizophrenic illnesses. The American Food and Drug Administration has in fact even agreed to include an 'anti-suicide' indication as part of the basis for prescribing clozapine. Further work is required in all areas of the management of schizophrenia, but the core point is that medication, effectively treating an individual's symptoms without unpleasant side-effects, is the essence of best treatment.

BOX 8.3   Medication and the course of schizophrenia

■ Patients treated in the pre-neuroleptic era (i.e. before the 1950s) show a much worse outcome overall

■ The longer the illness is left untreated, the less effective medication will be in reducing symptoms

■ A longer pre-treatment illness leads to more admissions and higher subsequent treatment costs

■ The longer treatment is delayed, the more relapses will occur and the longer will be the time to remission (i.e. recovery is slower)

■ Those patients who stop their medication have a very high relapse rate compared with those who do not, particularly if the medication is stopped abruptly rather than gradually

■ Trials of low-dose medication or 'intermittent targeted therapy' (i.e. on-off, as required if in a crisis) show significantly higher relapse rates

■ All the evidence shows that antipsychotic medication is the most effective means of preventing relapse in schizophrenia

---

 PATIENT QUESTIONS

8.27   Do I really need to 'keep taking the tablets' (Box 8.3)?

Many patients, despite what seems to be the best treatment in terms of medication and personal support, have ongoing illnesses. This can be a real curse, interfering with concentration, sleep and day-to-day activities in a general way. Nevertheless, without medication the situation would be much worse (see Q. 8.23), and it is important to have a clear grasp of what might happen to you if you stop. Most doctors would say that all patients should continue with their medication for at least the next 3–5 years, after which matters can be reviewed. Possible alternatives, how the medication is working, the (hopefully) social stability and any side-effects will all be part of that discussion, and both patient and carer (as well as professional) may realize that continuing with treatment is a good thing.

If continuing treatment means 'for life', comparisons have to be made with other chronic illnesses that are successfully treated by ongoing medication. These include diabetes (insulin injections, sometimes twice a day), thyroid failure (requiring regular thyroxine supplements), bronchitis and heart disease (both requiring a range of regular medications, for example to maintain cardiopulmonary function).

8.28 Are my voices just going to get worse and worse?

It is well-known that 'voices' – that is to say 'auditory hallucinations' – tend to be persistent. Some patients can learn to distract themselves and minimize the impact of these, whereas others suffer from them constantly and complain about this. All this may occur despite taking regular medication of the most appropriate type.

There is, however, evidence that many patients 'mellow out' over the course of time, most individuals tending to get no worse, and often to improve, beyond the 5-year mark. Despite having continuing symptoms, these become less distressing, you find you can learn new skills to distract yourself, and your behaviour becomes more settled because you do not feel so dominated by the symptoms. This is really the natural course of the illness, although ongoing medication is vital. Furthermore, it is often possible, with help, to turn unpleasant and derogatory voices into friendly companions, forms of cognitive therapy being increasingly sophisticated in terms of such developments. The Hearing Voices network has been particularly popular and effective in this area.

Conclusions and future prospects

9

9.1 How effective really are all our modern treatments compared with good social and family care?

There is no doubt that coming from a stable family background, with good social support, is a positive prognostic factor. No matter how caring the family, though, the great majority of patients require continuing medication. It is very much the *combination* of medication and a stable personal and social environment that provides the best outcome. The much improved lifestyle and ongoing mental state of patients with schizophrenia seen today is a tribute to this biopsychosocial approach. However, the lesson of history is that, without modern drugs, we would not have moved out of the asylums.

9.2 Is genetic research likely to help with future treatments?

Uncovering the human genome, alongside more specific genetic studies (e.g. into families with a strong family history of schizophrenia), is constantly strengthening our knowledge of the hereditary nature of schizophrenia.

Abnormalities on chromosome 1 have, for example, been linked to schizophrenia (and other mental illnesses) in a large Scottish family study, whereas an association with velocardiofacial syndrome (VCFS) implicates deletions on chromosome 22, and patients with VCFS have a high rate of schizophrenia. The hope for gene modification as part of treatment, as in other illnesses, remains, however, most uncertain. An established 'vulnerability' gene could, perhaps, help us better understand other precipitating factors and possibly generate specific vaccinations (e.g. to prevent a particular form of virus affecting a vulnerable person). A more worrying concern would be that prenatal genetic diagnosis could lead to considerable arguments, as well as family discomfort, related to the ethics of proceeding to pregnancy.

9.3 Are there any new forms of psychological therapy being developed?

Over the past three or four decades, psychological therapy has moved on in leaps and bounds, not least thanks to a more scientific approach to structuring treatment and measuring outcome. From the psychoanalytic tradition have developed a number of shorter approaches, for example cognitive-analytic therapy, combining aspects of both cognitive theory and analytical insight. The developments of behaviour therapy into cognitive-behavioural therapy, the use of short programmes of approximately 6–12 sessions and using specialized groups have also been helpful. The most obvious need at present, however, is for a sufficient number of properly trained clinical psychologists who can take on this work, at both the primary and secondary levels. Training programmes and refresher training programmes are also required for front-line nurses, whether in terms of anger management, anxiety management or motivational interviewing (for those with addiction problems.[16]

9.4 What new drug treatments will be available soon?

This has always been a big question, but several developments do seem to be nearly complete. A particular class of drugs called 'dopamine stabilizers' are emerging that do not just block dopamine – leading to unpleasant side effects – but also put the dopamine back in balance in its role in the brain's general neurochemistry. Research is also active in terms of looking at other parts of the brain's chemistry, for example drugs acting on glutamate or gamma-aminobutyric acid, both of which show potential abnormalities in some patients (*Box 9.1*).

BOX 9.1 Some new drug treatments?

Whereas modern drugs affect a range of brain neuroreceptors (e.g. acetyl choline or noradrenaline), their effects on dopamine (DA) and/or serotonin (hydroxytryptamine, 5HT) seem most important in treating schizophrenia. New 'atypical' antipsychotics, aimed in particular at reducing side-effects, include the following:

Aripiprazole	This seems to work as a dopamine stabilizer, stimulating presynaptic DA receptors but blocking post-synaptic ones. Minimal side-effects in terms of weight gain, abnormal or extrapyramidal movements, and ECG changes have been reported
Iloperidone	This acts at 5HT and DA receptors as an antagonist (i.e. blocking them). Again, a low incidence of weight gain and extrapyramidal side-effects has been reported so far. A depot preparation is also being developed
Ziprasidone	Mainly affecting 5HT receptors as an antagonist (i.e. blocking them), this has likewise shown a low incidence of weight gain and extrapyramidal side-effects. It is already available in some countries (available also as a short-acting intramuscular injection)

9.5 Are there any other forms of drug treatment in the pipeline that might be of benefit?

A particular need is for injectible forms of atypical drugs, and those for short-acting ones (olanzapine and ziprasidone) are already available. Depot preparations of atypical agents have been more difficult to develop, but the relatively unique Risperdal Consta, using a microcapsule formula, has been shown to be as effective as oral risperidone. This wider range of formulations – oral, injectible and long-acting injectible (depot) – will certainly enhance treatment options, and there is even talk of nasal sprays (*see Box 9.1*).

9.6 Might brain scans and/or surgery have something to offer in the future?

The localization of brain areas associated with particular schizophrenic symptoms is illustrated in *Figure 9.1*. The much more accurate techniques for prefrontal leucotomy – not commonly used in the UK but still effective for a few individuals – may in time have much to offer. Isolating specific lesions, for example in the temporal lobe, using new diagnostic techniques could generate subtle neurosurgical approaches to specific symptoms. The possibility of implants – such as those being employed for Parkinson's disease – should also not be ignored. Even the measurement of cerebrospinal fluid levels of neurochemicals in different parts of the brain may become standard practice.

9.7 Can we diagnose schizophrenia in the growing fetus?

This is not yet possible, nor has genetic research yet reached the stage of being able to predict that a particular individual's offspring will have the condition. Likewise, there is no evidence that any particular fetal abnormality has been associated with schizophrenia (although *see Q. 9.2* for the association between schizophrenia and VCFS) in terms of cerebral development or any other inherited abnormality. The likelihood of making such diagnoses in the future, however – as with, for example, Huntington's Chorea – will lead to considerable ethical difficulties.

9.8 What will be the likely impact of the new NHS Plan and specialist teams?

The details of the new NHS Plan for the UK, and the specialist teams involved in particular (Assertive Outreach, Crisis Intervention and Early Intervention) are outlined in *Box 9.2*. Such teams are seen as the vehicle whereby new government funding can be targeted to those in particular need in the mental health field. It is also planned to strengthen psychological treatment resources in primary care, with specific mental

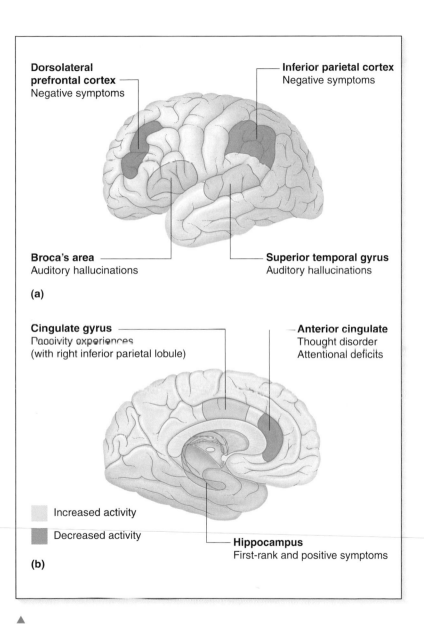

Fig. 9.1 The localization of brain areas associated with particular schizophrenic symptoms: (a) lateral view, (b) medial view of left hemisphere

---

BOX 9.2 2001 National Health Service Plan for Mental Health

	Primary care	Attached psychologists (>1000 newly recruited) + Primary care mental health teams Early Intervention Team (for first-onset/adolescent patients with schizophrenia)
Crisis Intervention and/or Home Treatment Teams	Community mental health team – multi-disciplinary, including nurses, social workers, psychiatrists, support workers and psychologists Assertive Outreach Team – as community mental health team but limited caseload, whole-team focus and specific interventions for hard-to-access patients	Acute inpatient psychiatric wards

---

health teams concentrating on the types of patient seen in primary care (who make up 80–90% of all those suffering with psychiatric problems). The needs of schizophrenic patients who are difficult to access, and those in the early stages of the illness, will be specifically addressed by Assertive Outreach and Early Intervention Teams respectively.

Concerns have been expressed about too many teams requiring too many interfaces and not having the staff to fill them. They may also tend to act as a magnet for the better, more enthusiastic staff, yet acute psychiatric wards, continuing care units and community mental health teams still have to provide most of the care. Balancing specialist resources with those generally responsible has led to criticisms that over-specialization is reducing the quality of care. Integrating and harnessing the enthusiasm and specialism of such approaches is going to be the challenge.

9.9   Is community care really effective in helping people with schizophrenia?

The evidence of community care being an effective form of treatment for people with schizophrenia is in fact quite robust. Despite the closure of most of the asylums and the fact that there are only about a fifth as many beds as there used to be 50 years ago (30 000 vs 150 000), the quiet successes of personal independence are everywhere to be seen. There has been no rise in the number of homicides carried out by mentally disordered individuals, and studies of patients discharged from the old asylums show 90–95% stability. Approximately 60–70% of patients with schizophrenia are living independently or semi-independently, and both patients and families have, in numerous research studies, expressed their preference for this kind of approach.

9.10   Is community care going to need a community treatment order?

Over the past 10 years, it has become clear that the effects of dual diagnosis – schizophrenia along with a drug or alcohol dependence problem – the funding shortages within the NHS, especially mental health services, and the lack of acute or rehabilitation beds for those who do relapse have all led to increasing concern. The rising tide of Sections of the Mental Health Act also seems to point to a difficulty in maintaining individuals without being able to resort to some kind of community treatment order. The arguments for and against such an approach are outlined in *Box 9.3*.

BOX 9.3   A community treatment order

Advantages	Problems
Ensures continuing care	Needs continuing medication
Avoids the 'revolving door' syndrome	Imposes treatment on those who are 'well'
Prioritizes 'difficult' patients	Perceived as intrusive social control
Reduces the stigma of regular relapse	Fears of 'kitchen-table' forcible injections
Maintains wellness rather than awaiting illness	Concerns about human rights and personal choice
Family and carers are reassured and supported	Evidence for effectiveness uncertain
Will enable more resources	?An alternative to proper community resources

9.11 Should we be thinking of rebuilding some form of asylum care?

Ever since the Inquiry into the care of Christopher Clunis (1994), which reported on the tragic death of Jonathan Zito on an underground station at the hands of Clunis, a relapsing patient with schizophrenia, there has been a rising tide of special reports highlighting just such 'untoward incidents'. These Inquiries – approximately 20 or more a year – tend to come out with very similar findings, for example the lack of resources, lack of communication and lack of coordination. The call to return to some kind of asylum care – and it is acknowledged that there are not enough long-stay or rehabilitation beds in the NHS – is naturally growing louder and louder.

In one sense, this is already happening, with a range of private and voluntary hostels and residences springing up all over the country. The private sector has been particularly active in this regard, and it is probably true to say that small is better. The original asylums were meant to house only about 30–50 people, then possibly 100–200, but ended up as barracks on hillsides with 3000 or more inmates. Their institutional deficiencies also emerged in a number of scathing reports into hospital scandals in the 1960s and 70s, so they are no panacea. The decline in bed numbers after 1980 has nevertheless accompanied a rise in Mental Health Act treatment orders (whereas both were gently decreasing together between 1955 and 1980), so we are probably short of medium- and high-dependence beds for those with a continuing illness. A return to large-scale institutions would. however, would be a real step back and likely to enhance stigmatization, public neglect and under-funding.

9.12 Is anything being done about the stigma of mental illness?

There is a very active anti-stigma campaign being led by the Royal College of Psychiatrists and supported by several pharmaceutical companies; a short film has been put out in cinemas, and it is now part of continuing policies. Particular approaches have included attempts at eliminating 'psycho' language from general discourse, in the same way as racist or ageist language is now no longer acceptable. Combined efforts with voluntary groups such as MIND or Rethink (formerly the National Schizophrenia Fellowship), and opposition to what is seen as the more stigmatizing aspects of the draft 2002 Mental Health Bill, are part of this approach. Continuing local initiatives in terms of education in schools, plays and documentaries on television or the radio, and the provision of services at the primary care level, along with other forms of medical treatment, should all have a positive effect. As with all such campaigns, it is likely to take a generation or two to remove the primitive fear of mental illness and its environment. The simple provision of small, purpose-built, attractive, modern facilities – rather than Victorian workhouses – for mental health patients and teams to operate from should in itself change psychiatry's negative image.

9.13 What are the current main research programmes in the UK in terms of schizophrenia?

These embrace a wide area of specialization, from detailed genetic studies through to high-contrast forms of brain scanning and studies into the psychology of schizophrenia. The effects of new medications on social and psychological functioning are regularly being reviewed, the Institute of Psychiatry (in south London) being one of the world leaders in such research. Useful websites are outlined in *Appendix 2*.

9.14 Where can I get more information about schizophrenia, particularly for families and carers?

There are numerous books, pamphlets and articles, in the lay and specialist press, that can give details about the illness. From the point of view of carers and patients, the most useful organizations are MIND, Rethink and Sane, whose telephone hotline 'Saneline' is readily available 24 hours a day (*see Appendix 2*). A number of recent books, suitable for people at all levels of education, are also summarized in *Appendix 2*. There is in fact such a mass of material that many carers and patients find it difficult to decide which might be most useful. Those included in Appendix 2 provide a combination of knowledge deriving from patients, their families and professionals, rather than one particular viewpoint.

9.15 What might a future schizophrenia treatment and care programme look like?

A future care programme would need to ensure early detection and treatment, continuing review and support, and help in terms of work and family. Thus, regular school age assessments, via specially trained teachers and educational psychologists, would identify those at risk. Sophisticated tests, whether brain scans or questionnaires, would enable a clear diagnosis as well as the setting up of a database of signs and symptoms against which one could monitor treatment. A local specialist treatment team – not stigmatized, thanks to educational and social initiatives – would take on patients and provide medication, personal therapy (whether cognitive, analytic or even more specific) and family education. This support would be automatic and easily transferable if people moved to another district. For patients still left with some degree of disability, working arrangements and jobs specially suited to their skills would enable them to have an independent income and lifestyle. Those with schizophrenia have a unique psychological make-up, and as new careers and skills emerge with the development of new technologies, it is hoped that those with schizophrenia will become as valuable in the workforce as the computer analysts who have taken up a new role over the past few decades.

BRIEF PSYCHIATRIC RATING SCALE (BPRS): ANCHORED

INFORMATION NOT OBTAINED ☐

Circle the degree of severity for each item:

Refer to the complete BPRS rating scale for a description of the items and the anchors

Degree of Severity

1 = Not present
2 = Very mild
3 = Moderate
4 = Moderately severe
6 = Severe
7 = Extremely severe
9 = Not assessed

Item									
1. Somatic concern	R	1	2	3	4	5	6	7	9
2. Anxiety	R	1	2	3	4	5	6	7	9
3. Emotional withdrawal	O	1	2	3	4	5	6	7	9
4. Conceptual disorganization	O	1	2	3	4	5	6	7	9
5. Guilt feelings	R	1	2	3	4	5	6	7	9
6. Tension	O	1	2	3	4	5	6	7	9
7. Mannerisms and posturing	O	1	2	3	4	5	6	7	9
8. Grandiosity	R	1	2	3	4	5	6	7	9
9. Depressive mood	R	1	2	3	4	5	6	7	9
10. Hostility	R	1	2	3	4	5	6	7	9
11. Suspiciousness	R	1	2	3	4	5	6	7	9
12. Hallucinatory behaviour	R	1	2	3	4	5	6	7	9
13. Motor retardation	O	1	2	3	4	5	6	7	9
14. Uncooperativeness	O	1	2	3	4	5	6	7	9
15. Unusual thought content	R	1	2	3	4	5	6	7	9
16. Blunted affect	O	1	2	3	4	5	6	7	9
17. Excitement	O	1	2	3	4	5	6	7	9
18. Disorientation	O	1	2	3	4	5	6	7	9

R = Reported / subjective information over approx. I week
O = Observed during the interview

Fig. A.1 Brief psychiatric rating scale (BPRS): anchored

APPENDIX 2
Useful websites and addresses

INFORMATION FOR PROFESSIONALS

British Association for Behavioural and Cognitive Psychotherapy
The website has a search facility for accredited therapists in your area, a list
of events and training provided by local branches, and a selection of leaflets
on topics including schizophrenia.
Website: http://www.babcp.org.uk/

British Psychological Society
For the register of chartered psychologists.
Website: http://www.bps.org.uk/index.cfm

Centre for Evidence Based Mental Health
An evidence-based mental health site.
Website: http://www.cebmh.com/

DSM criteria
Website: http://www.psychnet-uk.com/dsm_iv/dsm_iv_index.htm

National Electronic Library of Mental Health
Information for professionals and patients. Professional information
includes a list of current research and clinical trials, with links, diagnostic
criteria and evidence-based treatment summaries.
Website: http://www.nelmh.org/

National Institute for Clinical Excellence
Guidelines and algorithms on core interventions in the treatment and
management of schizophrenia in primary and secondary care issued
(December 2002) to the NHS in England and Wales.
Website: http://www.nice.org.uk/pdf/CG1NICEguideline.pdf;
http://www.nice.org.uk/pdf/CG1NICEguidelineoster.pdf

National Institute of Mental Health (NIMH)
Website: http://www.nimh.nih.gov/publicat/schizmenu.cfm

National Institute of Mental Health in England (NIMHE)
Part of the Modernisation Agency at the Department of Health. Their
website includes an archive of policy and frameworks, an events calendar

and details of NIMHE initiatives.
Website: http://www.nimhe.org.uk/

National Service Framework/National Guidelines
Website: http://www.doh.gov.uk/nsf/mentalhealth.htm

Primary Care Mental Health Education (PriMHE)
A non-profit-making organization that aims to help primary healthcare
professionals deliver the best standards of mental health care in various
ways, including educational and training initiatives, the fostering and
sharing of best practice, encouraging research and development, and
establishing collaborative and supportive partnerships with all concerned
organizations.
PriMHE
The Old Stables
2a Laurel Avenue
Twickenham
Middlesex TW1 4JA
Tel: +44 (0) 20 8891 6593 (administrative queries only)
Fax: +44 (0) 20 8891 6729
Website: http://www.primhe.org/

Royal College of Psychiatrists
Provides a brief overview of condition and points to the sources of further
help (some of which are included in this list).
Royal College of Psychiatrists
17 Belgrave Square
London SW1X 8PG
Tel: +44 (0) 20 7235 2351
Fax: +44 (0) 20 7245 1231
Email: rcpsych@rcpsych.ac.uk
Website: http://www.rcpsych.ac.uk/info/help/anxiety/

Journal articles
Collection of recent articles in the *British Medical Journal*.
Website: http://bmj.com/cgi/collection/schizophrenia

Evidence-based mental health journal.
Website: http://ebmh.bmjjournals.com/

Schizophrenia research

Highland Psychiatric Research Foundation
A research group investigating the 'phospholipid spectrum disorder' concept in the diagnosis and potential treatment of neurodevelopmental disorders, particularly schizophrenia.
Highland Psychiatric Research Foundation
Ness House
Dochfour Business Centre
Inverness IV3 8GY
Tel: +44 (0) 1463 220407
Email: info@hprf.org.uk
Website: http://www.hprf.org.uk/Research.html

Johns Hopkins School of Medicine
Collaborative research information on the genetics of schizophrenia and bipolar disorder.
Website: http://www.hopkinsmedicine.org/epigen/

Neuroscience Institute of Schizophrenia and Allied Disorders (NISAD)
Maintains a database of schizophrenia research projects currently planned or underway in New South Wales and the ACT, and offers people with schizophrenia the opportunity to register themselves as interested in becoming involved via a volunteer database of people who want to help.
NISAD
384 Victoria Street
Darlinghurst NSW 2010
Australia
Tel: +61 2 9295 8407
Fax: +61 2 9295 8415
Email: nisad@nisad.org.au
Website: http://www.nisad.org.au/about/index.html

Schizophrenia Research Foundation (India)
Non-governmental, non-profit-making organization in Chennai, India, which has since 1984 committed itself to schizophrenia research, education and patient care.
Schizophrenia Research Foundation (India)
R-7A North Main Road
AnnaNagar West (Extn.)
Chennai 600 101
Tamil Nadu, India
Tel: +91 044 6263971/6207073
Email: scarf@vsnl.com
Website: http://scarfindia.org/home.htm

INFORMATION AND SOURCES OF SUPPORT FOR PATIENTS

General mental health

Breakthrough

A service user-led research and training organization in mental health. It publishes a bi-monthly magazine, *Breakthrough*, produced by survivors of mental health and their carers.

Breakthrough
8 Trevelyan Place,
High Farm,
Crook,
County Durham DL15 9UY
Tel: +44 (0) 1388 767 404

Connects

A free linking website for mental health in general.
Website: http://www.Connects.org.uk

Internet mental health

A Canadian site of links to resources on various disorders – details include diagnosis, description (European and US), recent research, booklets and links to external sources of information.
Website: http://www.mentalhealth.com/

Jewish Association for the Mentally Ill

Offers guidance, counselling and support to sufferers and carers.
Jewish Association for the Mentally Ill
16a North End Road,
London NW11 7PH
Tel: +44 (0) 20 8458 2223
Website: http://www.mentalhealth-jami.org.uk

Mental After Care Association (MACA)

Provides information and services to people with mental health needs and their carers. MACA is active in the community, in hospitals and in prisons.
MACA
25 Bedford Square
London WC1B 3HW
Tel: +44 (0) 207 436 6194
Fax: +44 (0) 207 637 1980
E-mail: maca-bs@maca.org.uk
Website: http://www.maca.org.uk/intro.htm

Mental Health Foundation
A UK charity working in mental health and learning disabilities.
Website: http://www.mentalhealth.org.uk
UK Office
7th Floor
83 Victoria Street
London SW1H 0HW
Tel: + 44 (0) 20 7802 0300
Fax: + 44 (0) 20 7802 0301
Email: mhf@mhf.org.uk

Scotland Office
5th Floor, Merchants House
30 George Square
Glasgow G2 1EG
Tel: + 44 (0) 141 572 0125
Fax + 44 (0) 141 572 0246
Email: scotland@mhf.org.uk

Mental help net
A US 'megasite'.
Website: http://mentalhelp.net/

Mind
Campaigns for rights and develops locally based services. Its national
information line covers all aspects of mental health, including legal matters
for service users, carers, family and friends, researchers, students, service
providers and the public. Mind publishes a bimonthly magazine and has a
free quarterly newsletter as well as many other publications.
Mind
Granta House
15-19 Broadway
Stratford
London E15 4BQ
Tel: + 44 (0) 20 8519 2122; information line: + 44 (0) 20 8522 1728 if you live
in Greater London or + 44 (0) 8457 660 163 if you live elsewhere (Mon,
Wed & Thur 9.15 a.m. – 4.45 p.m.)
Email: contact@mind.org.uk
Website: http:// www.mind.org.uk

Samaritans
A UK Helpline for anyone experiencing emotional distress, providing
someone to talk to in confidence 24 hours a day. Details of local branches

can be found in the local telephone directory.
Samaritans
10 The Grove
Slough
Berkshire SL1 1QP
Tel: National helpline + 44 (0) 345 909090
Website: http:// www.samaritans.org.uk

SANE
A campaigning mental health charity. SANELINE, the helpline, gives information and support to anyone coping with mental illness.
SANE
2nd Floor
Worthington House
199–205 Old Marylebone Road
London NW1 5QP
Tel: + 44 (0) 20 7375 1002 (office); Saneline: + 44 (0) 845 767 8000 (open from 12 noon until 2 a.m. every day of the year)
Website: http://www.sane.org.uk

Scottish Association for Mental Health
Provides an information service and leaflets on general mental health issues.
Scottish Association for Mental Health
Cumbrae House
15 Carlton Court
Glasgow G5 9JP
Tel: +44 (0) 141 568 7000
E-mail: enquire@samh.org.uk
Website: http:// www.samh.org.uk

Threshold Women's Mental Health Initiative
A Brighton-based local services and a national information line run by and for women.
Threshold Women's Mental Health Initiative
14 St Georges Place
Brighton BN1 4GB
Tel: +44 (0) 845 300 0911; local rate 2–5 p.m. Mon–Thur
Website: http://www.thresholdwomen.org.uk/

Information and support for schizophrenia
Hearing voices network
A self-help network set up to help people who hear voices to find their own ways of coming to terms with their experience.

Hearing Voices Network
91 Oldham Street
Manchester M4 1LW
Tel: +44 (0) 161 834 5768
Email: hearingvoices@care4free.net
Website: http://www.hearing-voices.org.uk/

Making Space
A charity for schizophrenia sufferers and their families in the North of
England that runs residential homes, supported flats, day centres and self-
help groups, and employs family support workers.
Making Space
46 Allen Street
Warrington
Cheshire WA2 7JB
Tel: +44 (0) 1925-571680
Website: http://www.comcare.dial.pipex.com/making_space/

National Schizophrenia Fellowship Scotland
An organization offering information and support for people with
schizophrenia and their families/carers.
National Schizophrenia Fellowship Scotland
Claremont House
130 East Claremont Street
Edinburgh EH7 4LB
Tel: +44 (0) 131 557 8969
Fax: +44 (0) 131 557 8968
Email: info@nsfscot.org.uk
Website: http://www.nsfscot.org.uk/

National Voices Forum
An ex-service user and survivor network within Rethink that describes itself
as 'UK user-led organisation run by mad people for mad people'. Offers
empowerment and support via several local groups around the UK, as well
as an annual national conference and a quarterly magazine, *Perceptions*,
made up of contributions from the membership.
Website: http://www.voicesforum.org.uk/

Outreach and Support in South London (OASIS)
A service offering advice and support for people who may be having
psychological problems. OASIS aims to help people at high risk to get their
life back on track by early diagnosis and intervention, and usually offers
consultation within GP practices rather than psychiatric outpatient clinics.

The service is restricted to Lambeth, South London.
Tel/fax: +44 (0) 20 7848 0952
Email: oasislondon@hotmail.com
Website: http://www.oasislondon.com/

Rethink (previously the National Schizophrenia Fellowship)
Provides services and support for families affected by mental illness in the
UK. Rethink runs more than 300 services (including home treatment,
advocacy and helplines) around England, Wales and Northern Ireland,
which give practical support to around 7500 people every day.
Rethink
Registered Office
28 Castle Street
Kingston-Upon-Thames
Surrey KT1 1SS
Tel: +44 (0) 20 8547 3937; national advice service: +44 (0) 20 8974 6814,
Mon, Wed & Fri 10 a.m. – 3 p.m., Tue & Thur 10 a.m. – 1 p.m.
Fax: 020 8547 3862
Email advice@rethink.org
Website: http://www.nsf.org.uk/

Schizophrenia Association of Great Britain
Offers help to anyone who needs schizophrenia information and support
(sufferers, relatives or friends of sufferers, and carers or medical workers). It
produces a twice-yearly newsletter and other publications.
Schizophrenia Association of Great Britain
Bryn Hyfryd
The Crescent
Bangor
Gwynedd LL57 2AG
Tel: +44 (0) 1248 354048
Fax: +44 (0) 1248.353659
Email: info@sagb.co.uk
Website: http://www.sagb.co.uk/

Schizophrenia Fellowship New South Wales
Runs support groups (including some for non-English speakers) and a
telephone information service. The organization has been involved in the
development of clinical practice guidelines for the NSW Department of
Health. People with schizophrenia are involved at all levels of decision-
making, leadership, consultation and the general work of the organization.
Schizophrenia Fellowship New South Wales
Locked Bag 5014

Gladesville
New South Wales 1675
Australia
Tel: +61 2 9879 2600
Fax: +61 2 9879 2699
Email: info@sfnsw.org.au
Website: http://www.sfnsw.webcentral.com.au/

Schizophrenia Fellowship New Zealand
A voluntary organization for support and education, coordinated via local branches.
Website: http://www.sfnat.org.nz/

Schizophrenia Ireland
Provides a range of information, support and professional services for its membership, the general public and other service providers, including local support groups for sufferers and relatives of sufferers, courses for families and counselling. The organization also runs a helpline and employment services.
Tel: helpline 1890 621 631 (Mon, Weds & Fri 12–4 p.m, Thur 10 p.m. – 2p.m, Tues 3.30–7.30 p.m.)
Email: infor@sirl.ie
Website: http://www.sirl.ie/

Schizophrenia Society of Canada
Schizophrenia Society of Canada
75 The Donway West
Suite 814
Don Mills
Ontario M3C 2E9
Canada
Tel: +1 416-445-8204
Email: info@schizophrenia.ca
Website: http://www.schizophrenia.ca/

World Fellowship for Schizophrenia and Allied Disorders
A worldwide international organization for sufferers and their families. Members and associates provide direct services, run self-help groups, conduct workshops, produce educational materials, arrange conferences, advocate for better treatment and appropriate services, manage research funds and thus influence government policies. Publications available include documents in English, Spanish and Russian.
World Fellowship for Schizophrenia and Allied Disorders

869 Yonge Street
Suite 104
Toronto
Ontario M4W 2H2
Canada
Tel: +1 416 961-2855
Fax: +1 416 961-1948
Email: info@world-schizophrenia.org
Website: www.world-schizophrenia.org

Zito Trust
A charity set up to work towards the reform of mental health policy and
law, to provide advice and support to victims of community care
breakdown, and to carry out relevant research into services for the severely
mentally ill and disordered. The Trust also works to raise awareness of the
need to ensure that patients with mental illness receive the new treatments
now available.
Zito Trust
16 Castle Street
Hay-on-Wye
Hereford HR3 5DF
Tel/Fax: +44 (0) 1497 820011
Email: zitotrust@btinternet.com
Website: http://www.zitotrust.co.uk/

Other web resources
http://www.chovil.com/
A personal website with various information and resources as well as
individual accounts of one man's experience of schizophrenia.

http://www.docguide.com/news/content.nsf/PatientResAllCateg/
Schizophrenia?OpenDocument
Summaries of the latest medical news and alerts, as well as more basic
information.

http://www.emental-health.com/schizophrenia.asp
Free registration to access the latest news and research, and discussion boards

http://www.openthedoors.com/
A site sponsored by the World Psychiatric Association. Information for
professionals and patients on schizophrenia, as well as a global programme
to advance knowledge and combat stigma. The site is accessible in several
languages.

http://www.schizophrenia.com/
A not-for-profit information site, including information and discussion boards.

Stigma and mental illness

http://www.sane.org/
StigmaWatch: an initiative by SANE Australia monitoring the media for inaccurate or discriminatory references to mental illness and encouraging journalists to be fairer and more accurate in how they report this area. SANE Australia also offers information, fact sheets and a helpline online.

http://www.stigma.org/
An organization working to support the destigmatization of mental illness along with a consortium of other initiatives, including Changing Minds, the campaign by the Royal College of Psychiatrists.

REFERENCES

1. World Health Organization 1973 Report of the international pilot study of schizophrenia. WHO, Geneva
2. Rosenhan D 1973 On being sane in insane places. Science 179:250–258
3. Dixon L, Haas G, Weiden P J et al 1991 Drug abuse in schizophrenic patients: clinical correlates and reasons for use. American Journal of Psychiatry 148(2).224–230
4. World Health Organization 1992 The ICD-10 classification of mental and behavioural disorders. Clinical descriptions and diagnostic guidelines. WHO, Geneva
5. World Health Organization 1979 Schizophrenia: an international follow-up. John Wiley, Chichester
6. Baron M 2001 Genetics of schizophrenia and the new millennium: progress and pitfalls. American Journal of Human Genetics 68:299–312
7. Crow T J 1983 Is schizophrenia an infectious disease? Lancet i:173–175
8. Fuller, T E 1980 Schizophrenia and civilisation. Aronson, New York
9. Zammit S, Allebeck P, Andreasson S et al 2002 Self-reported cannabis use as a risk factor for schizophrenia in Swedish conscripts of 1969: historical cohort study. British Medical Journal 325:1199–1201
10. Retterstøl N 1987 Present state of reactive psychosis in Scandinavia. Psychopathology 20:68–71
11. Taylor P J, Gunn J 1999 Homicides by people with mental illness: myth and reality. British Journal of Psychiatry 174:9–14
12. Szmukler G 2000 Homicide inquiries – what sense do they make? Psychiatric Bulletin 24:6–10
13. Wessely S 1997 The epidemiology of crime, violence and schizophrenia. British Journal of Psychiatry 170 (supplement 32):8–11
13. Cookson J, Taylor D, Katona C 2002 Use of drugs in psychiatry, 5th edn. Gaskell/Royal College of Psychiatrists, London
14. National Institute for Clinical Excellence 2002 Schizophrenia – clinical guidelines I, December 2002. NICE, London
15. Vaughn C E, Leff J P 1976 The influence of family and social factors on the course of psychiatric illness: a comparison of schizophrenia and depressed neurotic patients. British Journal of Psychiatry 129:125–137
16. Turkington D, Kingdon D 2000 Cognitive-behavioural techniques for general psychiatrists in the management of patients with psychoses. British Journal of Psychiatry 177:101–106

FURTHER READING

Adolescents

Clark A F 2001 Proposed treatment for adolescent psychoses. I: Schizophrenia and schizophrenia-like psychoses. Advances in Psychiatric Treatment 7(1):16–23

Advance directives

Papageorgiou A, King M, Janmohamed A et al 2002 Advance directives for patients compulsorily admitted to hospital with serious mental illness. Randomised controlled trial. British Journal of Psychiatry 181:513–519

Clinical symptoms

Gelder M, Mayou R, Cowen P 2001 Schizophrenia and schizophrenia-like disorders. In: Shorter Oxford textbook of psychiatry, Oxford University Press, Oxford, Ch12, pp 329–377

Gelder M, Mayou R, Cowen P 2001 Paranoid symptoms and paranoid disorders. In: Shorter Oxford textbook of psychiatry. Oxford University Press, Oxford, Ch13, pp 381–397

Turner T H 1998 Schizophrenia. In: Davies T, and Craig T K J (eds) ABC of mental health. BMJ Books, London, pp 27–31

Community care

Bennet D H, Freeman H L (eds) 1991 Community psychiatry. The principles. Churchill Livingstone, Edinburgh

Guest L, Burns T. 2001 Community care for patients with schizophrenia – a UK perspective. Journal of Advances in Schizophrenia and Brain Research 3(2): 34–42

Drug treatments

Crow T J, MacMillan J F, Johnson A L et al 1986 A randomised control trial of prophylactic neuroleptic treatment. British Journal of Psychiatry 148:120–127

Geddes J, Freemantle N, Harrison P et al 2000 Atypical antipsychotics in the treatment of schizophrenia: systematic overview and meta-regression analysis. British Medical Journal 321:1371–1376

Kane J, Honigfeld G, Singer J et al 1998 Clozapine for the treatment-resistant schizophrenic: a double-blind comparison with chlorpromazine. Archives of General Psychiatry 45:789–796

Reveley M A, Deakin J F W 2000 The psychopharmacology of schizophrenia. Oxford University Press, New York

Epidemiology

Sartorius N, Jablensky A, Korten A et al 1986 Early manifestations and first-contact incidence of schizophrenia in different cultures. Psychological Medicine 16:909–928

Shepherd M, Watt D, Falloon I et al 1989 The natural history of schizophrenia: a 5 year follow up study of outcome prediction in a representative sample of schizophrenics. Psychological Medicine Monographs 15 (supplement):1–46

For patients and carers

Hemmings G 1989 Inside schizophrenia – a new comprehensive guide for sufferers and their families. Sidgwick & Jackson, London

Torrey E Fuller 1995 Surviving schizophrenia – a family manual. Harper Collins, New York

Wilkinson G, Kendrick T 1996 A carer's guide to schizophrenia. Royal Society of Medicine, London

General

Andrews G, Jenkins R (eds) 1999 Management of mental disorders, vol 2, UK edn. WHO Collaborating Centre for Mental Health and Substance Abuse, London

Johnstone E, Humphreys M S, Lang F H, Lawrie S M, Sandler R 1999 Schizophrenia – concepts and clinical management. Cambridge University Press, Cambridge

Mortimer A, Spence S 2001 Managing negative symptoms of schizophrenia. Science Press, London

Stefan M, Travis M, Murray R M 2002 An atlas of schizophrenia. Parthenon, London

Stein G, Wilkinson G (eds) 1998 Seminars in general adult psychiatry, vol 1. Gaskell/Royal College of Psychiatrists, London

History

Shorter E 1997 A history of psychiatry from the era of the asylum to the age of Prozac. Wiley & Sons, New York

Psychological treatments

Wykes T, Tarrier N, Lewis S (eds) 1998 Outcome and innovation in psychological treatment of schizophrenia. John Wiley, Chichester

Rating scales

Andreasen N C, Olsen S 1982 Negative and positive schizophrenia. Definition and validation. Archives of General Psychiatry 39(7):789–794

Farmer A, McGuffin P, Williams J 2002 Measuring psychopathology. Oxford University Press, Oxford

Overall J E, Gorham D R 1962 The Brief Psychiatric Rating Scale (BPRS). Psychological Reports 10:799–812

Wing J K, Cooper J E, Sartorius N 1974 The measurement and classification of psychiatric symptoms. Cambridge University Press, Cambridge

GLOSSARY

Anhedonia – The term used to describe the inability to enjoy things, in particular or in general. It is the opposite of hedonism (i.e. pleasure-seeking) and is regarded as a typical, negative, symptom of schizophrenia.

Bipolar psychosis – Also known as bipolar affective disorder. This is a modern term to describe manic depressive disorder. Such illnesses vary between the two 'poles' of being very high/manic to being very low/depressed. It is used to form a contrast with patients who suffer from only one type of condition (unipolar), that is to say those who are only either depressed *or* manic.

Passivity experience – An important 'first-rank' symptom of schizophrenia and regarded as one of the 'positive' symptoms of that condition. It describes the state of patients not being in active control of their thoughts, feelings or movements, such that they feel these are imposed upon them by something or someone from outside. They are thus the passive recipients of actions, which is often a frightening and intrusive experience.

Psychomotor retardation/poverty – Describes the state of those who are slowed down in the way in which they think, speak and move. It is commonly part of a severe depressive illness but can also be seen in forms of schizophrenia, such as catatonic schizophrenia. It is literally as if patients are living the experience of a 'slow motion' film.

Schizoid – Describes personalities who are introspective, rather cold and detached towards others, who prefer being on their own and who seem rather indifferent to the world outside. They are often perfunctory and limited in their communication with others, tend to be humourless but may spend their time just thinking about some aspect of philosophy or religion. Something resembling schizoid traits may precede the onset of full schizophrenia, but the majority of individuals just go on being schizoid.

Schizotypal – Describes personalities who are somewhat odd in their beliefs and rather suspicious of others, tend to be a bit eccentric, rarely have any close friends and show considerable social anxiety. They often feel estranged and out of touch, and the condition seems to be genetically related to schizophrenia, with an increased incidence in the families of schizophrenic patients.

Schnauzkrampf ('snout spasm') – A German term describing the tendency of some patients with schizophrenia, especially catatonic schizophrenia, to wrinkle their nose and thrust their rounded lips forward in a tubular fashion. This resembles an animal's snout and is regarded as a form of stereotyped behaviour, a disordered form of expression. It is less common than in the days before medication was available as symptoms are now treated effectively.

Thought broadcast – Describes the first-rank symptom of experiencing one's thoughts being broadcast out and known to those around one. It is as if other people know what you are thinking, is similar to the notion of telepathy (i.e. mind-reading) and is often perceived as intrusive and frightening.

Thought disorder – Describes the difficulty that many patients have in organizing their thoughts, in following a consistent train of thought and in expressing their thoughts clearly. Speech is often hesitant, muddled and difficult to follow. Severe forms take on a kind of 'word salad', language being jumbled up into a completely incomprehensible pattern.

LIST OF PATIENT QUESTIONS

INDEX

Note: As Schizophrenia is the subject of the book, all index entries refer to schizophrenia unless otherwise indicated. Page numbers in **bold** type refer to figures or tables. Cross references in *italics* indicated general references (e.g. *see also specific agents*).

A

U

V

W

Y

Z